E Tai Chi

(THE BASIC BOOK)

The World's Simplest Tai Chi

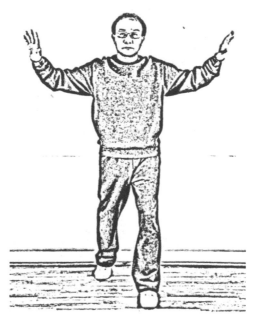

Invented, Written, and Demonstrated by

Yongxin Li, M.D., Ph.D.
Internal Medicine Physician

Copyright

E Tai Chi
(The Basic Book)

The World's Simplest Tai Chi

First Edition: November 2016
(Updated: January 2019)

ISBN-13: 978-0692800669
ISBN-10: 0692800662

E Tai Chi Logo

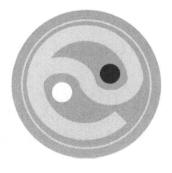

This book is dedicated to:

My wife, Jo, who is my first E Tai Chi student;
My children, Jason and Megan, who are my hope;
Dad, Shanquan, who said to me, "You won't achieve anything if you don't keep fit."

****
****

Also by Dr. Yongxin Li

Life and Medicine

E Tai Chi
(The Basic Book-Chinese Edition)

E Tai Chi
(The Complete Book)

Yoga E Tai Chi
(The Basic Book)
At Amazon.com

Yoga E Tai Chi
(The Advanced Book)

E Tai Chi
(The Science Book)
Coming soon.

E Tai Chi Song

Learning simple Tai Chi is so easy,
Walking sideways won't hurt your knee,
Qigong exercises reduce stress,
Versatile workouts benefit you infinitely.

Things are never perfect,
Life is short and hectic.
Let's practice E Tai Chi,
Keep fit and be cheery.

By Yongxin Li

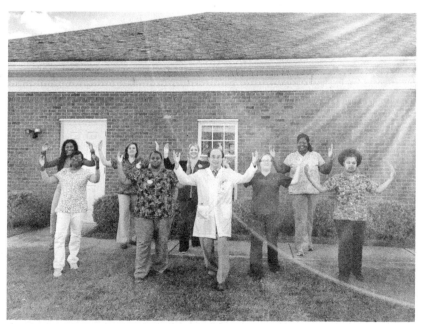

Practicing E Tai Chi during break times.

Educational Disclaimer

The medicine and E Tai Chi described in this book can be viewed as common medical knowledge and a guide to exercises. The movements or postures in E Tai Chi are scientifically designed and have been applied to my patients safely. Since they involve only gentle hand/arm movements and normal walking or standing, they should not pose a greater risk of injury than people's normal daily activities do. Nevertheless, any exercise can cause potential injuries. You should consult a qualified medical professional before starting a new exercise such as **E Tai Chi**. The author disclaims any and all liability for damages resulting from the use of information in this book.

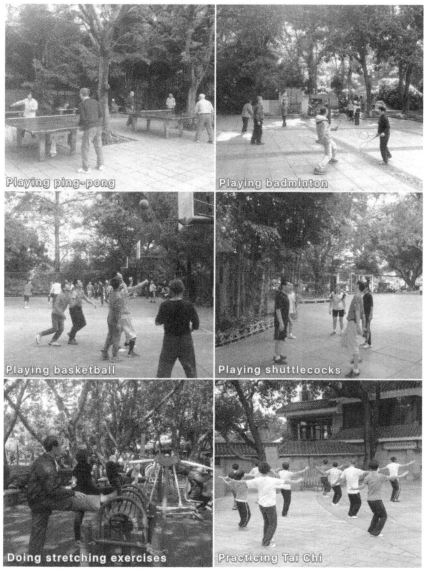

Various outdoor exercises in China.

Practicing Tai Chi is just one of the many morning exercises Chinese people do in the park.

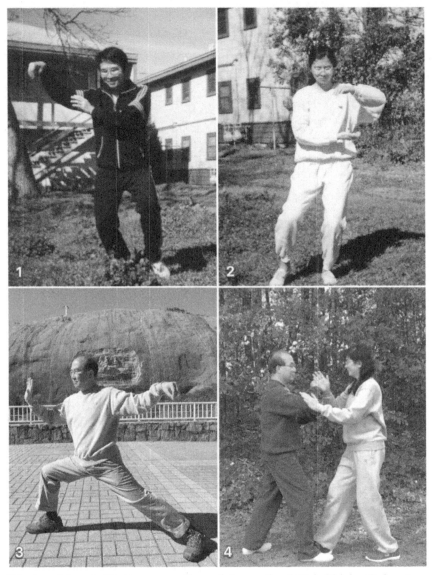

Photos #1 and **#2**: Jo, my wife and I practiced Tai Chi in Galveston, Texas, in 1986.

Photos #3 and **#4**: Today, three decades later, Tai Chi remains one of our favorite exercises.

Table of Contents

Prolog

Travelers, there is no path, paths are made by walking.

—Antonio Machado (1875-1939, Spanish Poet)

Tai Chi is also known as **Tai Chi Chuan** or **Taijiquan**, one form of Chinese martial arts, which is characterized by its tranquility, slowness, relaxation, smoothness, and continuity. It is a combination of physical and mental exercises and has been proven to provide many health benefits, e.g., reducing stress, preventing falls, and improving some chronic medical disorders including hypertension, depression, fibromyalgia, and other chronic pain conditions.

E Tai Chi (**Ease** or **Easy Tai Chi**) is the world's simplest and safest **Tai Chi** exercise, which is invented by Dr. Yongxin Li, a practicing physician with a Ph. D. degree in physiology. It consists of sequences of simple and gentle circular hand/arm movements performed with normal walking or standing.

E Tai Chi is unique, original, scientific, effective, and infinite! Its characteristics can be summarized by Five S's: **Simplicity**, **Science**, **Safety**, **Strength**, and **Serenity**.

Simplicity. E Tai Chi is the ultimate simplest Tai Chi, which cannot be simplified any more. Besides regular standing or walking, E Tai Chi is made of only **one** circular hand/arm movement, which gives rise to **six** basic movements readily. E Tai Chi can be learned without an instructor. You can learn how to practice basic standing and walking E Tai Chi within minutes. You can master the basic E Tai Chi sequence within an hour or its whole sequence within two to three days by reading this book and watching the accompanying illustrations and videos.

Science. E Tai Chi is an entirely brand-new Tai Chi exercise system that is scientifically created for the purpose of simplicity, safety, and efficacy. It is not the rearrangement or modification of existing Tai Chi

Forms. E Tai Chi is the essence of Tai Chi extracted from traditional Tai Chi and maintains the beauty of Tai Chi without its shortcomings such as being difficult to learn, causing joint injuries, etc. There are only six basic hand/arm movements in E Tai Chi. Except for the movement, **Cloud Hands** that is present in all the current Tai Chi styles, the remaining five movements are completely newly designed. You can execute these movements vertically, horizontally, in any circular manner, and with any combinations of vertical and horizontal performances.

Safety. The typical Tai Chi walk, the curved footwork, has been replaced by regular walking or slowed natural walking in E Tai Chi. You always face forward without making turns, squatting, or kicking. Because you walk sideways in most of the E Tai Chi postures, you can avoid over-flexion of the knees and maintain optimal knee-foot alignment. All these safety designs will minimize injuries induced by Tai Chi exercises. You can practice E Tai Chi safely anywhere, anytime, during normal walking, and in any position (sitting, standing, or even lying). Thanks to its gentle arm/hand movements and regular standing or walking, E Tai Chi is safe, especially for older people.

Strength. In the E Tai Chi sequence, the majority of the postures involve walking sideways. E Tai Chi provides an efficient physical workout because sideways walking consumes over three times more energy than forward walking. You can tone up your muscles by performing E Tai Chi with weights on your wrists. Moreover, you may even turn E Tai Chi into an aerobic exercise if you practice it at a fast pace.

Serenity. E Tai Chi combines Tai Chi with **Qigong**, a Chinese style body-mind exercise. This integration will enhance the efficacy of Tai Chi exercises.

You can create your own E Tai Chi sequence by using the six basic hand movements and different ways of walking or standing. The six hand/arm movements can be transformed further into any movements of existing Tai Chi styles. Therefore, E Tai Chi has laid a solid foundation for you if you wish to pursue traditional Tai Chi forms in the future.

E Tai Chi relaxes your body, reduces stress, promotes physical fitness, and cultivates the sensation of feeling good. Since E Tai Chi is simple and safe, you can easily incorporate it into your day to day life. If you want to practice Tai Chi and Qigong to improve your health, then E Tai Chi is the only Tai Chi and Qigong you need for the rest of your life.

In this book, I have tried to focus on teaching how to learn E Tai Chi quickly and to perform it safely as opposed to discussing the mysterious and unscientific theories about traditional Tai Chi, Qigong, and Chinese Medicine. People that are interested in those theories can read other Tai Chi and Qigong books. Also, you can learn about my views of Chinese medicine in my book (*Life and Medicine, Chapter 6, Seeing Doctors in China*). By using common sense, we know that any moderate, safe, and regular exercise will have health benefits. In the 21st century, what we need is science, peace, prosperity, and health.

I use at least nine photos to illustrate each E Tai Chi movement or each walking step in E Tai Chi sequences. These photos, many of which are the images extracted from the video recordings, provide detailed and genuine demonstrations of the E Tai Chi exercises. The e-book version also contains video recordings of all the E Tai Chi movements, postures, and complete E Tai Chi sequences.

In order to make the learning process simple and not to overwhelm the readers with numerous figures and instructions, I publish two books about E Tai Chi: the basic book and the complete book. The complete book of E Tai Chi covers the intermediate and advanced E Tai Chi plus the majority of the contents of the basic book. Tai Chi beginners can read the basic book first. They can study the complete book when they have become familiar with the basic E Tai Chi.

The complete book with over 900 photos contains much more color images than any other Tai Chi or Qigong books on the market.

Recommended Study Plan

Level One E Tai Chi (two to three hours)

1. Learn Movements 1, 2, and 3.
2. Perform them while standing and walking.
3. Learn the basic sequence (five postures).

Level Two E Tai Chi (one to two days)

1. Learn Movements 1 to 6.

2. Perform them while standing and walking.

3. Learn the intermediate sequence (ten postures).

Level Three E Tai Chi (You can reach the advanced level almost spontaneously after having become proficient in practicing Level Two E Tai Chi.)

1. All above.

2. The advanced sequence. Perform the same ten postures as in the intermediate sequence but in a different way.

List of Video Recordings

(These videos are embedded in the Kindle eBook version of the book.)

Complete Basic E Tai Chi Sequence (Page 50)

Complete Basic E Tai Chi Sequence (Page 116)

Movements 1, 2, and 3 (Page 81)

Starting Posture and Posture One (Page 121)

Posture Two and Posture Three (Page 135)

Posture Four (Page 147)

Posture Five (Page 157)

Closing Posture (Page 162)

Basic E Tai Chi Performed Vertically and Horizontally (Page 165)

Also, you can watch the videos of E Tai Chi sequences demonstrated by the author on YouTube:

E Tai Chi (the introduction)

https://www.youtube.com/watch?v=8SpGNjAtxPw

E Tai Chi (the basic sequence)

https://www.youtube.com/watch?v=QjbVILwHwCY

E Tai Chi (the intermediate and advanced sequences)

https://www.youtube.com/watch?v=Medo50cBNEc

Introduction

Live life in harmony and balance. Avoid excesses. Even good things, pursued or attained without moderation, can become a source of misery and suffering.

—M. A. Soupios and Panos Mourdoukoutas
(Authors of *The Ten Golden Rules: Ancient Wisdom from the Greek Philosophers on Living the Good Life*) (Mourdoukoutas, 2012)

The first man that ever ran the marathon (around 26 miles) in 490 BC, Pheidippides, collapsed and died immediately after he reached his destination. Human beings were not designed for prolonged intensive aerobic exercises, and they have a storage of glycogen that provides energy only for 30 km/18-20 miles of running. (For more details on this topic, see *Wikipedia: Marathon.*) However, people hold more than five hundred marathons all over the world every year. Amateur marathon runners continue to be exposed to the marathon-induced harmful effects such as heart disorders, electrolyte imbalance, muscle and joint injuries, etc. Although I respect and admire the spirit of the marathon, I dislike the actual marathon running that poses health risks. Moderation in all things is the key.

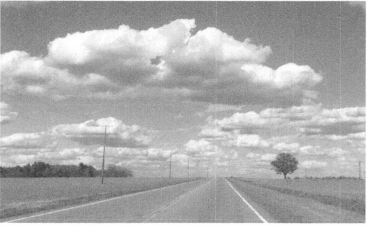

Questions?

Why do I need to invent or create a new Tai Chi exercise since so many Tai Chi styles have already existed?

Why am I qualified to do this kind of work?

Why is E Tai Chi an invention?

Why is this new Tai Chi style, E Tai Chi, an excellent exercise for your body and mind?

When I entered the exam room, I found that Mr. Young, in his 40s, was standing with his hand holding the edge of the exam table painfully.

"Why are you standing, Mr. Young?" I asked.

"Doc, I am in trouble," he replied. "My back hurts like hell."

"What's happened? Lifting something heavy or a fall?"

"No. I went to a Yoga class last night. I was okay then. However, when I woke up this morning, I cannot move my back at all. There is so much pain in the lower back that I cannot sit down. I feel less pain when standing up."

"I guess you have developed back injury probably due to overstretching during the Yoga class."

"Please help me get rid of the pain, Doc."

The patient was one of the many yoga-induced injury cases I had encountered during the first few months after I started my new job in this town in 2013. For example, a woman complained about hip and groin pain after a few months' Yoga exercises. A middle-aged man developed severe abdominal wall pain because of over-bending his body during a Yoga session. A young Yoga learner came in with a limping leg, complaining of leg pain with numbness of her foot and toes.

A couple of years ago, a patient of mine even collapsed while performing Yoga neck bending in the gym. She was sent to the ER by an ambulance. Fortunately, she had recovered completely without sequela.

Of course, many other patients come to see me because they suffer from a variety of musculoskeletal disorders after running, doing weightlifting, playing tennis or basketball or golf, etc. Unquestionably, all sports and physical exercises potentially cause injuries, especially in older people.

"I don't think you have a severe spinal injury," I said to Mr. Young after a physical exam. "I will prescribe some muscle relaxants and pain pills for you. Hopefully, you'll get better in a week or so."

"What next?"

"Stay away from Yoga for a few weeks or forever."

"I like the mental exercise in Yoga. What can I do in the future if I can't do Yoga?"

"You can try Tai Chi. I think Tai Chi is another exercise that combines physical and mental workouts."

I showed him some Tai Chi performances on YouTube on the computer screen. I usually let my patients watch the 24-Form Simplified Tai Chi. Gao Jiamin's performance is always on the top list on YouTube.

"She is playing so smoothly and elegantly. She looks beautiful too," Mr. Young said.

"Sure, she is beautiful! However, you need to know she is a Chinese Tai Chi champion. You cannot imitate her long strides and high kicks. Those movements cause injuries as Yoga does. The athletes do these for a living like NBA players, who frequently check in to the orthopedic clinics and have their knees fixed during the off-season."

"I like it very much. How can I learn it?"

"You can buy a book with DVD or watch YouTube videos."

"I got a Tai Chi video some years ago. But it is too difficult to learn on my own. And I can't find a Tai Chi teacher around this area."

Many friends and patients told me that they bought books and tapes or discs for Tai Chi. However, they could not learn Tai Chi from those materials and gave it up eventually. All their Tai Chi books and discs are covered with dust on the bookshelf.

As the saying goes, "Learn to walk before you run." When it comes to Tai Chi learning, people tend to do the opposite. The most mysterious and unscientific thing I can think of about the contemporary Tai Chi is that almost all the Tai Chi forms have complicated beginning movements. Even in the Simplified 24 Form, you need to make a turn before you can go on to the next posture after finishing the **Commence** posture. What is the point of putting some complicated movements in the beginning postures of each Tai Chi sequence? These challenging starting postures scare away many potential Tai Chi learners.

Most of the Tai Chi books on the market are not easy to follow, especially without an instructor. Even some of the authors state in their books that one cannot learn Tai Chi by reading their books. Many Tai Chi books emphasize "**qi**" and "**dantian**," which have never been proved to be real scientifically. They are the old concepts of traditional Chinese Medicine, which are the primitive understanding of nature by the ancient people. The imaginary qi and dantian make Tai Chi more mysterious and harder to learn.

Furthermore, Tai Chi learners and practitioners tend to flex their knees too much. Over-flexion of knees may damage knee joints. The whole body weight is supported by only one leg in many postures. It is not safe for older people to perform those Tai Chi postures, which may cause joint injuries and falls.

As I work 10-12 hours daily and on some weekends, I cannot do any actual Tai Chi teaching. Over the past few years, I have been thinking of designing a Tai Chi form everybody can learn without an instructor and perform anywhere, anytime without injury. Finally, E Tai Chi has been created and introduced in the book.

Why am I qualified to write this book?

1. I have 44 years of experience practicing Chinese martial arts.

2. I can practice all the popular Tai Chi forms: 24-Form, 48-Form, 42-Form, Yang, Wu, Hao (Wu), Chen, Sun, and Zhaobao styles. I can perform them not only traditionally from right to left but also in the opposite direction, from left to right. I have learned many prevalent Qigong exercises.

3. I used to be a scientist with a Ph.D. degree and have a good knowledge of the structures and functions of the human body.

4. I am a practicing primary care physician, talking with patients about physical exercises daily and understanding how different sports affect them.

5. I came to the U.S. at the age of 31. I know how to read classic Chinese books on Tai Chi, Qigong, and traditional Chinese medicine (TCM). I am familiar with Chinese and English medical literature on Tai Chi studies.

6. I have collected and read more than one thousand Tai Chi and Qigong books in both Chinese and English.

E Tai Chi is entirely distinct from the current Tai Chi styles. It is a style of simplicity and safety. Tai Chi learners can learn E Tai Chi just by reading my book with accompanying videos. Moreover, it takes just hours or days to master it!

I believe **E Tai Chi** is the world's simplest and safest Tai Chi, which maintains the beauty of traditional Tai Chi and makes the best use of the health benefits of Tai Chi without injuries. E Tai Chi focuses on health benefits, and it does not care about the so-called "Tai Chi fighting skills," which are misleading, impractical, and even dangerous.

E Tai Chi is simple because it consists of only **one** circular hand/arm movement and regular walking or standing. This single circular movement straightforwardly evolves into six basic hand/arm movements, which can be learned within two to three hours. Additionally, the hand/arm movements are symmetrical in most circumstances (except Movement 6, see Chapter 4 in the complete book). When you learn to perform E Tai Chi by reading this book, you do not need to reverse the Tai Chi movements in the pictures. Of course, I provide many lateral views of various postures. Therefore, you can see how all the postures or movements are performed at different angles.

You always face forward without making turns. Turning around can be dangerous to older people. You can learn E Tai Chi without an instructor.

E Tai Chi is safe because it is composed of gentle hand/arm movements and regular walking or standing. Indeed, one can trip and fall even when taking a normal walk, particularly in the case of senior citizens. Nevertheless, this is life! We all need to be careful whenever we do something in our life.

All the Tai Chi styles except Chen style consist of no more than 40 different movements or forms. Some people do not consider Chen Style as a typical or standard Tai Chi exercise because it contains many abrupt and strenuous movements, which do not fit the characteristics of Tai Chi: smoothness, relaxation, and fluidity. It seems that no one has created a new style of Tai Chi since Wu style Tai Chi was designed eight decades ago. For example, the latest style of Tai Chi, Dongyue Taijiquan (东岳 太极), was crafted by Professor Men Huifeng (门惠丰教授）in 2000 (Men 门, 2011). However, none of its movements or postures is newly designed. Namely, Dongyue Tai Chi is a sequence of Tai Chi forms that were chosen from the existing styles of Tai Chi and put together.

E Tai Chi is an invention because it is not a rearrangement or modifications of existing Tai Chi forms. It is a brand-new Tai Chi exercise system. Even though the six hand/arm movements in E Tai Chi look straightforward and familiar, five of them excluding **Cloud Hands** have never been seen before in all styles of Tai Chi. For example, all the current Tai Chi styles have Cloud Hands, but nobody has thought that Cloud Hands can be "reversed" to become **Reverse Cloud Hands**. Cloud Hands is executed **vertically** with **sideways walking** or standing in all the styles of Tai Chi. Has anyone imagined that Cloud Hands can be implemented **horizontally** or while walking **forward** or **backward**? In fact, you can take any direction you like when performing Cloud Hands in E Tai Chi. Furthermore, you can wave your hands in large or small circles because there is no strict rule in E Tai Chi. The only rule is easy, which means simple, safe, and gentle.

Even though these five movements are newly designed, they are derived from the essence of existing Tai Chi. Most importantly, they are easy to learn and safe to practice. Also, I get rid of unhealthy curved Tai Chi walk, jumps, kicks, Half Squat Stance (*pubu*), etc. I use regular walking or standing instead.

Thus, E Tai Chi is easy to learn, and one can practice it safely anywhere and anytime. Once one has learned the basic skills, he or she can improve continuously. The one basic movement can develop into various graceful movements, which can be performed while walking forward, backward, or sideways. Furthermore, you can play them as slowly or as fast as you want while sitting, standing, walking, and even lying in bed.

It helps reduce stress, maintain balance, prevent falls, and alleviate neck, back, and shoulder pain. It promotes relaxation physically and mentally. You can increase muscular strength by performing faster movements or holding weights (physically) and meditate by slow movements coordinated with breathing (mentally).

Naturally, it takes weeks or months to improve your smoothness, continuity, and relaxation. However, you can build up your confidence right away by mastering E Tai Chi within minutes or hours. Since you can learn how to perform and enjoy E Tai Chi on the first day, you will practice it daily from that moment on and achieve its health benefits. If you are young and physically fit, you can go on to learn any types of traditional Tai Chi after picking up E Tai Chi.

I have been showing E Tai Chi to some of my patients during office visits. They can learn it within five minutes. Some patients say that they forget it when they go home. Therefore, I decided to write a simple book everyone can use at home.

This is the only book from which you can learn Tai Chi by yourself. It contains more detailed illustrations than any Tai Chi books on the market. Most of the tai chi books place flowcharts at the end of a chapter or a book. Therefore, learners do not know where to walk. In contrast, in this book, the systematic flowcharts are placed at the beginning of posture-teaching. They show where you go, how many steps you walk, and how you move your feet.

You do not have to face the west or the east when you practice E Tai Chi. There is no scientific evidence that facing the east is healthier than facing the west or the north or south. In E Tai Chi, you can walk in any direction or even walk circularly.

I try to provide front views and lateral views of each posture and detailed explanations of the transitions of postures, which are the most difficult to learn. Some of the descriptions, illustrations, and flowcharts are repeated in some sections so that you can have a complete instruction for each movement without reference to other chapters.

In this book, I have tried to focus on teaching how to learn E Tai Chi quickly and to perform it safely as opposed to discussing the mysterious and unscientific theories about traditional Tai Chi, Qigong, and Chinese Medicine. People that are interested in those theories can read other Tai Chi books.

Chapter 1 briefly describes the concept and history of traditional Tai Chi, its shortcomings, and its health benefits.

Chapter 2 addresses the characteristics of E Tai Chi and its advantages.

Chapter 3 introduces the basics of E Tai Chi.

Chapter 4 illustrates the six hand/arm movements in E Tai Chi.

Chapter 5 describes practicing E Tai Chi with regular standing and walking.

Chapter 6 teaches the basic E Tai Chi sequence.

Chapter 1. Demystifying Tai Chi

《题西林壁》
横看成岭侧成峰，远近高低各不同。
不识庐山真面目，只缘身在此山中。

Written on the Wall at West Forest Temple
From the side, a whole range; from the end, a single peak:
Far, near, high, low, no two parts alike.
Why can't I tell the true shape of Lu-shan (Mount Lu)?
Because I myself am in the mountain.

—苏轼 (Su Shi, 1037-1101, Chinese Poet)
Translated by Burton Watson

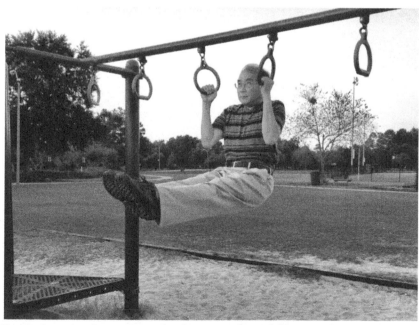

Doing hanging leg raises remains one of my daily exercises

The above poem implies that *lookers-on see most of the game*. I have never had a formal Tai Chi teacher. I started to learn some Tai Chi postures from a co-worker more than 40 years ago when I was working at a printing factory in China. Since then, I have studied Tai Chi just from reading books, watching videotapes, videodisks, and observing people practice in the parks in China. Of course, I enjoy watching beautiful Tai Chi performances on YouTube and other Chinese video websites such as 56.com, youku.com, etc.

Since I do not claim to be a student or disciple of any Tai Chi master, I do not have the burden of keeping any one's style. Tai Chi is simply my hobby, and I am good at it. As I do not teach or conduct research on Tai Chi for a living, I have no conflict of interests related to Tai Chi. What I have is science, modern medicine, and clinical experience. I create E Tai Chi and write a book about it for the purpose of helping my patients. Certainly, the book will benefit other people who are interested in simple and safe Tai Chi. That is to say, I am entirely an outsider to the field of Tai Chi. Hence, I am able to look at Tai Chi exercises from a different perspective.

What Is Tai Chi?

Tai Chi is an abbreviation of Tai Chi Chuan or Taijiquan. **Tai Chi (Taiji, 太极)** means the origin of the universe, "supreme ultimate," in Chinese, which is not related to martial arts. Here **Chuan** or **Quan** (拳) means "fist or boxing" in Chinese. I will use Tai Chi in most circumstances in this book because I dislike anything implying "fighting." (For more details on this topic, see *Wikipedia: Tai chi.*)

Tai Chi, one type of Chinese martial arts, is characterized by its tranquility, slowness, relaxation, smoothness, and continuity. It is a combination of physical and mental exercises. Chinese martial arts (wushu，武术) have been existing for thousands of years. They are merely individual or personal fighting skills and have nothing to do with real wars in Chinese history. Although Tai Chi masters emphasize its fighting techniques, Tai Chi has never been proved to be a practical fighting skill even in one to one fighting, and never played any role in battlefields. A famous Chinese general, Qi Jiguang (戚继光, 1528－1588), wrote several hundred years ago, "Learning a martial art is for enhancing physical fitness only, not for fighting in battlefields." Numerous anecdotes tell that prominent Tai Chi masters could throw away opponents without bodily contact. Yet, no one has ever been able to demonstrate this type of technique in front of a camera.

In the West, boxing is purely a fighting sport. On the contrary, Tai Chi, the most popular Chinese martial art, has been incorporated into Chinese culture, sports, and entertainments. There have been dozens of martial art movies that depict the mysterious, "superior" Tai Chi fighting. Overemphasizing its combat aspect will be misleading, impractical, and even dangerous in the 21st century.

Many Tai Chi books claim that Tai Chi is a great treasure of China's cultural heritage. However, most Chinese people did not know the existence of Tai Chi until the Chinese government started to promote it in the 1950s and 1960s. Tai Chi has never played any significant role in eliminating diseases, promoting population health, bringing prosperity, and repelling invaders in Chinese history.

In summary, Tai Chi can be considered to be one of the many exercises or sports that improve **personal** health. Nevertheless, Tai Chi is unique because it emphasizes both physical and mental training. Most importantly, Tai Chi is a safe exercise or sport (Wayne, et al., 2014). It has been scientifically proven to have many health benefits (Hempel, et al., 2014). It not only helps to improve some medical disorders but also cultivates the sensation of feeling good through its slow, smooth, relaxed movements. This gentle and comfortable exercise is particularly suitable for older people.

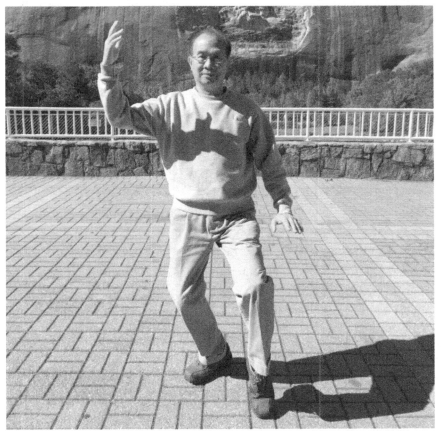

White Crane Spread Its Wings in traditional Tai Chi.

A Brief History of Tai Chi

The origin of Tai Chi is still controversial. However, Zhang Sanfeng (张三丰，in the 12th century?), a legendary Taoist, is commonly considered as the creator of Tai Chi. But there were several Taoists known as Zhang Sanfeng. Tai Chi was initially practiced by Taoists or monks secretly. Most books state that a businessman named Wang Zhongyue (王宗岳, in the 15th Century?) happened to learn Tai Chi from someone (a Taoist?). Then he taught Tai Chi techniques to Zhang Fa (张发, in the 15th century?), who lived and learned Tai Chi in Wang's home for seven years. Zhang Fa started to teach Tai Chi when he came back to his hometown, Wen County, Henan Province, China. It is debatable who Zhang Fa's first student was. At least, it has been well documented that people in the area started to practice Tai Chi four hundred years ago. (For more details on this topic, see *Wikipedia: Tai chi.*)

Until the late 1800s, Tai Chi had been practiced for several hundred years only by small groups of individuals like monks, some martial art teachers, and their dedicated students. The majority of Tai Chi practitioners and learners lived in Henan Province, China, during that time. The story tells that Yang Lushan (杨露禅，1799-1872) went to Chen Village, Henan Province, and stayed there many years learning Tai Chi. Yang Lushan returned home and then went to Beijing, the capital city of China, to teach Tai Chi. Since then, Tai Chi has spread out to other parts of China over the next 100 years and then to many other countries over the past 50-60 years.

Tai Chi is hard to learn. There is a saying, "It takes ten years to master Tai Chi." Some great teachers, such as Yang Chengfu (杨澄甫, 1883-1936) had tried to simplify Tai Chi and created Yang style Tai Chi, which is easier to learn. Tai Chi masters have created many different styles of Tai Chi. There are six most popular Tai Chi styles as follows:

Yang style Tai Chi is the most popular one that was simplified and standardized by Yang Chengfu (杨澄甫).

27

Chen style Tai Chi is commonly considered as the oldest Tai Chi originated in Chen Village, Henan Province. The creator of Yang style Tai Chi lived and studied Tai Chi in the village.

Zhaobao style Tai Chi has existed for a long time like Chen style Tai Chi. Some people think that Chen style Tai Chi is derived from Zhaobao Tai Chi, which is the original Tai Chi created by Zhang Sanfeng, the legendary creator of Tai Chi.

The other prevalent styles include Wu, Hao (Wu), and Sun. They were all rooted in Yang style. (For more details on this topic, see *Wikipedia: Tai chi*.)

Finally, the Chinese government organized Tai Chi experts to design the 24-Form Simplified Tai Chi in 1955. The government had also trained thousands of instructors to teach 24-From for free in China. As a result, millions of people can practice 24-Form in China. Since then, 48-Form, 42-Form, 88-Form Yang Tai Chi have been designed by the government sports committee. Later on, the Competition Forms of Yang, Chen, Wu, Hao (Wu), and Sun styles have come into being.

All these government-designed Tai Chi exercises are simply the rearrangements and minor modifications of the traditional Tai Chi forms. Nonetheless, their movements, forms, or postures have been standardized and scientifically designed to be more symmetrical and become easier to learn. Many Tai Chi teachers have immigrated or traveled to other countries and taught Tai Chi for the past several decades. It is estimated that there are more than one hundred million Tai Chi practitioners and learners all over the world.

The Health Benefits of Tai Chi

Tai Chi is a unique exercise that combines physical and mental training. Any moderate and safe exercise can make you live better and longer (Lear, Gasevic, & Hu, 2016). Simplicity and moderation are everything in life. One should never do anything excessively. You do not have to exert yourself to the utmost or stretch your body immensely to achieve the health effect of an exercise or sport. Practicing Tai Chi can offer some specific health benefits without serious injuries (Hempel, et al., 2014).

In my opinion, Tai Chi can promote health mainly in two areas, reducing stress and improve musculoskeletal functions. Stress is related to almost all common chronic diseases, including coronary artery disease, hypertension, stroke, diabetes, mental disorders such as depression, anxiety, etc. Slow and relaxing Tai Chi movements help people become more relaxed and distracted from their stresses. As the stress level is lowered, these chronic disorders such as hypertension and depression can be improved or even eliminated.

Tai Chi has been proven to alleviate musculoskeletal pain and stiffness, improve gait balance, reduce falls in senior citizens or patients with Parkinson's disease, and speed up recovery from a stroke. A recent review by VA has summarized the evidence of Tai Chi potential benefits in hypertension, depression, falls, balance confidence, osteoarthritis, pain, COPD, muscle strength, and cognitive performance (Hempel, et al., 2014).

Tai Chi and Yoga emphasize both physical and mental exercises. When compared with Tai Chi, yoga is harder to learn and tends to have a higher risk of inducing injuries. Yoga is a strenuous exercise that requires active stretching. It has been reported that Yoga can cause various injuries, including sprains, strains, dislocations, fractures, ligamentous or muscle tears, and even strokes. It leads to many emergency room visits yearly in the U.S. Even some yoga teachers suffer themselves (Penman, M, P, & S, 2012) (Broad, 2012).

In contrast, Tai Chi is much more gentle, relaxed, and smooth with fewer adverse effects (Wayne, et al., 2014). Tai Chi is a dynamic exercise requiring walking while yoga is a static exercise without moving around. **E Tai Chi** is even more versatile because you can practice dynamically (walking) or statically (standing).

Although practicing Tai Chi provides many health benefits, **Tai Chi is not a panacea**. It does not cure HIV, treat Ebola, or get rid of polio. I can guarantee that it does not cure or prevent hair loss. Yang Chengpu (杨澄甫, the creator of Yang style Tai Chi), was bald in his 40s according to his photos. (If you want to look at his picture, see *Wikipedia: Tai chi.*) So am I. Certainly, Tai Chi cannot cure cancer. But it may improve the quality of life in patients with cancer (Zeng, Luo, Xie, Huang, & Cheng, 2014).

This book is intended to show you how to practice E Tai Chi. If you want to know more about the health benefits of Tai Chi, you can refer to Wikipedia and the references in this book or read the book by Dr. Peter Wayne (Wayne & Fuerst, 2013).

The Shortcomings of Existing Tai Chi

Although the modern Tai Chi forms have their standardized movements and postures, they are only the rearrangement and minor modification of the traditional Tai Chi styles and cannot get rid of the shortcomings of the traditional Tai Chi. For example, they are still difficult to learn, especially for non-Chinese.

All the Tai Chi styles except the 24-Form Tai Chi have some complicated beginning movements including **Grasp the Bird's Tail** or **Lazy about Tying Coat**. Notably, even the **Commencing** postures in Chen style and Zhaobao style Tai Chi are challenging to learn. I am not sure if Tai Chi masters intended to drive Tai Chi learners away or to impress their students. Anyhow, Tai Chi students have to spend weeks or months studying these several movements even if they do not quit.

All the Tai Chi books on the market are difficult to follow, esp. without an instructor. Even some of the authors state in their books that one cannot learn Tai Chi by reading their books. Some of the Tai Chi movements are too challenging for ordinary people to learn, e.g., **Lotus Kicks** and **Half Squat Stance** in almost all the Tai Chi styles. How many regular Tai Chi learners can perform **Dragon Dives to the Ground** (雀地龙) in Chen style Tai Chi? This posture is not only

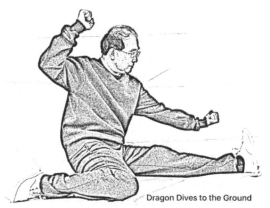

Dragon Dives to the Ground

difficult to learn but also harmful to joints. Furthermore, it cannot be a practical fighting technique either.

Many Tai Chi books pay too much attention to fighting applications when teaching Tai Chi movements. Some books state that you cannot master real Tai Chi if you do not know the martial applications of each posture. Few people learn Tai Chi for the purpose of fighting or even self-defense. That will make it harder to learn Tai Chi. In my opinion, you will grasp the real meaning of Tai Chi when you have completely forgotten its fighting techniques and power. Then you will become peaceful and relaxed and achieve its health benefits.

It has not been reported that amateur Tai Chi learners suffer a stroke or severe neck/back injuries because of practicing Tai Chi. Here, I am not talking about professional Tai Chi athletes. They jump or kick as high as possible and squat as low as possible. Remember that you do not imitate the leg movements of Tai Chi masters on DVD or YouTube. They are professionals, athletes, and champions, who do these performances for a living, but not for health purposes. They entertain us with those beautiful and challenging acrobatic movements, which have nothing to do with promoting health.

Even though Tai Chi does not cause serious adverse effects such as fatal or life-threatening events, it can induce overuse injury to joints. The most common disorder caused by Tai Chi is knee pain or injury. Interestingly, in the west, some studies indicate that practicing Tai Chi can alleviate knee pain (Wang, et al., 2016) (Yan, et al., 2013) (Nahin, Boineau, Khalsa, Stussman, & Weber, 2016). The majority of the Tai Chi studies did not mention adverse effects caused by practicing Tai Chi (Wayne, et al., 2014). In a recent study on the effect of Tai Chi on knee osteoarthritis, the authors reported no serious adverse events such as fatal, life-threatening, incapacitating events, hospitalizations, etc. without mentioning anything about worsening knee pain (Wang, et al., 2016). Surprisingly, it seems that all the participants in the Tai Chi and physical therapy groups had achieved beneficial effects on their knees (Wang, et al., 2016). Nevertheless, no medical treatment modality is free of adverse effects. In my clinical practice, my patients tell me from time to time that knee treatments with physical therapy, steroid injection, or even knee surgery make their knee pain worse.

On the contrary, Tai Chi induced knee pain and injury are widespread in China (Zhu, et al., 2011). A recent survey found that more than 50 percent of Tai Chi practitioners reported knee pain after practicing Tai

Chi (Yuan 苑, 2014). Tai Chi-induced knee pain has become a hot topic in the Tai Chi community and got its nickname "Tai Chi Knee (太极膝)." Numerous studies and articles on this subject have been published in China. You can do a google search if you are interested in this issue.

Many Tai Chi students tend to over-flex their knee joints because a lot of Tai Chi teachers and professional athletes practice Tai Chi this way. You can watch their performances on YouTube. For example, the image of **Outdoor practice in Beijing's Temple of Heaven** on Wikipedia shows a Tai Chi practitioner (the man wearing a white shirt and black pants in the center of the picture), whose front knee is over-flexed and protrudes over the toes even though his stance is high. If you want to look at the image, see *Wikipedia: Tai chi*.

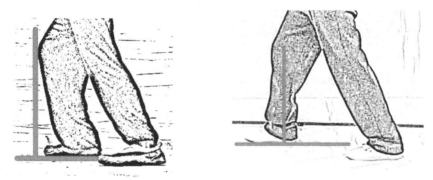

Figure 1-4A. Knee flexion in a bow stance. Left: Incorrect Stance. The front knee protrudes over the toes of the foot. Right: Correct Stance. Ideally, the front leg should be perpendicular to the foot or ground.

Taking a low stance and long strides will place even more strain on the knees and other joints, leading to not only knee but also ankle and hip injuries. Life is contradictory. Delicious food is usually unhealthy. Similarly, the long stride and low stance look beautiful but are harmful to joints, especially knee joints.

In many styles of existing Tai Chi including 24-Form, practitioners cannot keep their knees aligned with the tips of their feet when making turns and rotating the torso because of some of the unhealthy Tai Chi postures. The abnormal twisting of the knees will cause knee injuries easily. For example, when you perform the first **Parting the Wild Horse's Mane** posture after finishing **Commencing** in 24-Form, you must step out to the left with your left foot while turning the torso left at the same time. Because the supporting knee (the right knee) is not in line with the tip of the foot, knee pain or injury is likely to occur. See **Figure 1-4B**.

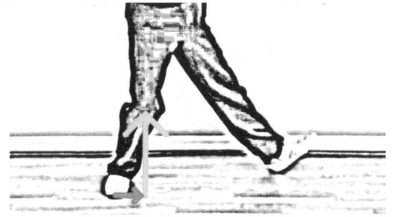

Figure 1-4B. The first Parting the Wild Horse's Mane posture in 24 Form Tai Chi. The supporting knee (the right knee) is not aligned with the tip of the foot.

In many postures of traditional Tai Chi, people are not supposed to move their steps straightforward, but in a curved route. First, they need

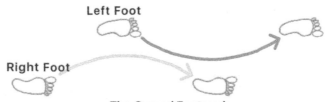

to rotate their legs to turn their torso and shift the body weight. Secondly, they move their swinging foot close to the standing foot and then shift it back to the original side. The rotation of the legs may twist the knee and ankle joints, and the supporting leg will carry the whole-body weight for an extended time. As a result, the knee and ankle joints will get hurt easily. The curved walking is especially unsafe for older people.

When it comes to "fighting," no real fighter would like to use Tai Chi footwork or curved walking in an actual fight, as has been demonstrated in modern-day fighting competitions such as Tai Chi sanshou, boxing, karate, and any other martial arts. All fighters adopt a natural stance with mildly flexed knee joints. Furthermore, there is no evidence that curved walking provides more health benefits than regular walking. Also, no martial art master takes a horse stance or a bow stance when carrying out a fight even in a movie.

For millions of years, human beings have used natural walking to carry out most of their activities. They have walked out of Africa and reached every corner of the world. Walking on foot differentiates us from other animals. Walking is the most natural way to move around. We need to keep walking for almost all our lives.

Why do we need a Tai Chi step or footwork that is harmful to joints? Is it because my teacher's teachers or my ancestors did this way? Sun style Tai Chi has the safest way to walk because the rear foot follows the front foot closely without loading the body weight on one leg for an extended period of time. Naturally, when people stand and wait in line, they tend to use one foot to support the body weight, the other foot lightly touching the ground for balance only. Unfortunately, the most popular Tai Chi, 24 Form, preserves the curved footwork.

All the traditional styles of Tai Chi except Chen Style are not aerobic exercises and do not increase upper extremity strength effectively even though all of them provide a lot of lower-extremity training. Of course, too much weight bearing would destroy the smoothness and relaxation of Tai Chi. Tai Chi is not a panacea. You need to do weight training if you want to build up muscles. Alternatively, you can speed up metabolism by running, playing tennis, etc.

Any moderate and safe physical exercises have health benefits and can make you live better and longer. Tai Chi is simply one of them. Most importantly, you exercise moderately, safely, and regularly.

Chapter 2. E Tai Chi

Sometimes the questions are complicated and the answers are simple.

—Dr. Seuss (1904-1991, American Author)

Walking is man's best medicine.

—Hippocrates (460–370 BC, Greek Physician, Father of Modern Medicine)

"The proverb says you do not need more than enough of anything. I have learned that moderation is the key to everything in life and medicine. One should never do anything excessively. Too much exercise may hurt your joints and even your heart, and excess eating can cause many diseases, including obesity and diabetes. Eating right and exercising judiciously will make you live better and longer." (Quoted from my book, *Life and Medicine*.)

E Tai Chi is a symbol of moderation and simplicity.

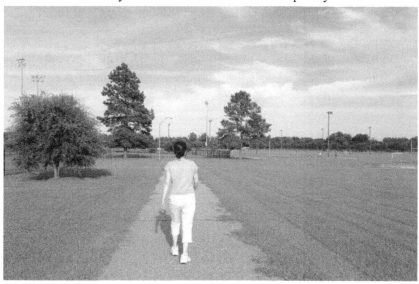

Taking a walk in the park.

The Characteristics of E Tai Chi

These days, **E**-anything is a cool name, such as e-mail, e-book, e-commerce, and even e-medicine. "E" in **E Tai Chi** is an abbreviation of "**Easy** or **Ease**," not "electronic." "Easy" or "ease" means simple, gentle, and comfortable. **E Tai Chi** is a style of simplicity, gentleness, and comfort.

I would like to compare E Tai Chi to **Metformin** (antidiabetic medication). Metformin, the treatment base for type 2 diabetes, is the most widely prescribed antidiabetic in the world. It has also been used in many other conditions, including polycystic ovarian syndrome, prevention of diabetes, weight control, adjunct cancer therapy, and even dementia.

Metformin originated from French Lilac. (See details in the section of Chapter 5: Diabetes-Metformin as Herbal Medicine in my book, *Life and Medicine*.) (Li, 2015) Scientists started to extract the active ingredients from French lilac in the 1800s. However, all those extracts that could lower blood sugar level in animals and humans turned out to be too toxic for clinical use. One of the extracts was scientifically modified to become a useful and safe drug, Metformin.

For the same reason, even though having health benefits, traditional Tai Chi has many shortcomings as described above. E Tai Chi is scientifically extracted and developed from the traditional Tai Chi. Through cautious modification and redesign, Tai Chi has become simple, easy to learn, and causes less or no injury from practicing it (with few or no adverse side effects).

E Tai Chi is a newly invented style of Tai Chi, which is entirely different from the current Tai Chi styles. E Tai Chi emphasizes simplicity, safety, and health benefits. It is for personal health only and has nothing to do with fighting or even self-defense. There are only six hand/arm movements in E Tai Chi. Except for **Cloud Hands** that exists in all the Tai Chi styles, the remaining five movements look straightforward, but they are entirely newly designed. Furthermore, the typical Tai Chi walk, catwalk, has replaced by regular walking or slowed natural walking. Therefore, I call it an invention.

In addition to maintaining all the health benefits of traditional Tai Chi, E Tai Chi has the following advantages, which can be summarized as the **Five S's**: **Simplicity, Science, Safety, Strength,** and **Serenity.**

Simplicity. As I mentioned previously, I have condensed all the current Tai Chi movements into only **one** circular movement. In biology, a cell is the basic structure of living organisms, the simplest unit of life except for viruses. Similarly, E Tai Chi is the Tai Chi exercise at the cellular level. Therefore, it cannot be simplified anymore if you want to maintain the essential characteristics of Tai Chi.

There are numerous hand/arm movements, stances, and kicks in traditional Tai Chi. Even in the book about standardized Tai Chi, Professor Li Deyin (李德印教授) introduces 33 hand/arm movements, 10 stances, 14 ways of walking, and 6 types of kicking (Li 李, 2003). In E Tai Chi, you perform **six** hand movements, **five** stances, and **three** ways of normal walking without kicking, squatting, or making turns.

In E Tai Chi, the single circular hand/arm movement gives rise to the **six** basic movements readily. The symmetry of its movements makes it easy to learn and remember. You can learn E Tai Chi without an instructor. Movements 1, 2, and 3 are so easy that everybody can learn them within minutes. If you perform them while standing or walking naturally, then you can say you have learned E Tai Chi.

Unlike traditional Tai Chi forms, Posture One is the simplest form at the beginning of the basic E Tai Chi sequence. The following Postures are as simple as Posture One. Movement 4 in E Tai Chi is the traditional **Cloud Hands (Wave Hands like Clouds)**. Although it is one of the most beautiful Tai Chi postures, most of the Tai Chi books describe it in a very complicated way. I do not think any Tai Chi beginner can learn how to perform Cloud Hands by reading those books. Here I can summarize Cloud Hands in **one** sentence: **Sequentially circle your hands in front of you while walking sideways or standing.**

Therefore, it just takes two to three hours to master the basic E Tai Chi. You have finished the learning process in E Tai Chi if you do not want to go any further. Late on, what you need to do is to practice, perfect, and enjoy it.

Science. E Tai Chi is a complete brand-new training system, which is scientifically designed according to the principles of simplicity, safety, and efficacy. It is not based on unscientific concepts such as Yin/Yang, meridians, Five Elements, imaginary organs, and so on.

As mentioned earlier, knee pain is a major injury due to practicing Tai Chi. A higher degree of knee flexion during Tai Chi practicing poses an increased risk of suffering Tai Chi-induced knee pain (Yuan 苑, 2014).

The normal gait cycle consists of eight phases: initial contact, loading response, midstance, terminal stance, preswing, initial swing, midswing, and terminal swing. The knee joints sustain the most weight load during the loading and mid-stance phases. The maximum knee flexion during the loading and midstance phases is 15-20 degrees (University of Washington) (Dicharry, 2010) (Rose, n.d.). The average walking step length is about 26.4 inches (67 cm) for women and 30 inches (76 cm) for men (The United States Department of Veterans Affairs).

Since walking is the safest and most effective exercise for human beings, I have tried to make the walking exercise in E Tai Chi as close to the natural walking as possible. I adopt the 15-20-degree flexion of knee joints in E Tai Chi **Routine Stance** (see Chapter 3) after reviewing a lot of scientific research on walking gait and Tai Chi exercises. However, the degree of knee flexion will be increased spontaneously when you practice slow normal walking in E Tai Chi sequences. I propose that the flexion of the knees should not be over 20-30 degrees, and the length of each step should be within 30 inches (76 cm) in order to prevent knee injuries. See **Figure 2-1A**. Also, the knee should always be kept in line with the tip of the foot.

You can practice E Tai Chi anywhere and anytime. You can perform the hand/arm movements in any direction, horizontally, diagonally, and vertically. The circular hand movements can be expanded and shrunk to achieve different exercise effects. Even though I illustrate the core principles of performing E Tai Chi, there is no strict rule. The rule is that you are doing right as long as you feel natural, comfortable, and painless.

E Tai Chi should not cause more pain even if you have knee pain before practicing it. If it is the case, you need to keep adjusting your stance with less flexion of knee joints and shorter steps until your knee pain returns to its baseline level. Alternatively, just walk naturally as usual.

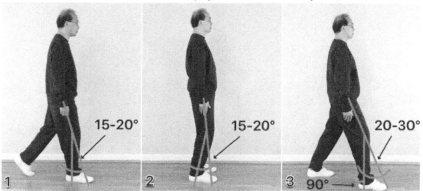

Figure 2-1A. Knee flexion during normal walking, in Routine Stance, and during slowing walking in E Tai Chi sequences.

Photo #1: Normal walking during the loading response phase. The knee joint reaches 15-20 degrees of peak flexion. The step length is about 2 feet (60 cm), which is comfortable for me.

Photo #2: Routine Stance. This stance is taken all the time when practicing E Tai Chi sequences.

Photo #3: Slow walking in E Tai Chi sequences. The degree of front knee flexion should be kept within 30 degrees. The front lower leg should be perpendicular to the ground, and the front knee should be aligned with the tip of the foot.

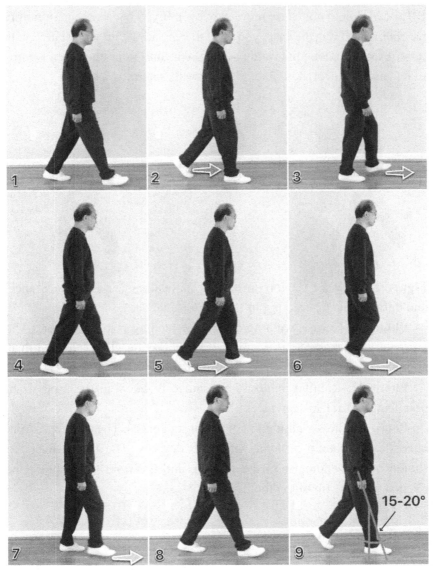

Figure 2-1B. Phases of gait during normal walking.

Key points for **Figure 2-1B**.

Photo #1: **Initial Contact.** The right foot is moving forward with the right heel hitting the ground.

Photo #2: **Loading Response**. Shift the body weight to the right leg with the entire right foot contacting the ground. Lift the left heel up and get ready to step forward with the left foot.

Photo #3: **Midstance**. The left foot is swinging forward.

Photo #4: **Terminal Stance**. The left heel touches the ground. Gradually shift the body weight to the left leg.

Photo #5: **Preswing**. As the body weight has moved entirely to the left leg, the right heel comes off the ground. You are ready to step forward with the right foot.

Photo #6: **Initial Swing**. The right foot is swinging forward and passing the left foot.

Photo #7: **Midswing**. The right foot continues to move forward.

Photo #8 (= Photo #1): **Terminal Swing**. The right heel hits the ground. Now you can repeat the same cycle of normal forward-walking.

Photo #9: The same as **Photo #2 (Loading Response)**. The peak flexion of the knee.

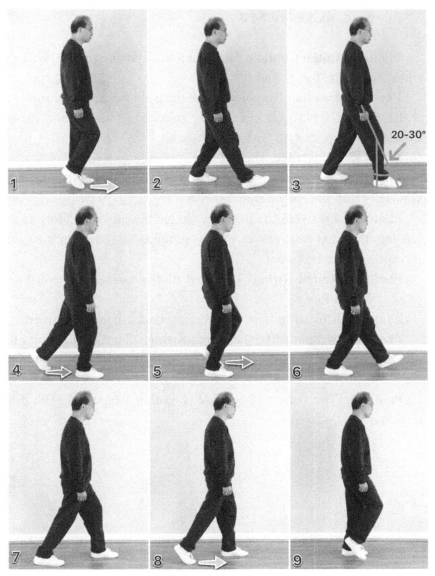

Figure 2-1C. Slow forward walking in E Tai Chi sequences.

Key points for **Figure 2-1C**.

Photo #1: This is **Transitional Stance**: one of the legs (the left leg in the figure) is supporting the body weight while the toes of the other leg (here the right leg) gently touch the ground to maintain balance.

Photo #2: Step forward with the right foot. The right heel comes in contact with the ground.

Photo #3: Gradually shift the body weight to the right leg. Now, you are in **Bow Stance**: your front knee (here the right knee) is mildly flexed with the back leg (here the left leg) straight. The degree of front knee flexion should be kept within 30 degrees. The front lower leg should be perpendicular to the ground, and the front knee should be aligned with the tip of the foot.

You should use the rear leg to push the body forward so that the front lower leg forms a 90-degree angle relative to the front foot or the ground. This is a standard **bow stance** in Chinese martial arts. When **you drive the body forward by the rear leg,** the front knee joint will not be over-flexed. That is the most critical measurement to prevent knee injuries. This principle applies to all the forward movements.

Photo #4: As the body weight is completely transferred to the right leg, the left heel comes off the ground. You are ready to swing the left leg forward.

Photo #5: The left leg swings forward until it becomes parallel to the right leg. The toes of the left foot gently touch the ground. Now you are back in **Transitional Stance**.

Photo #6: Step forward with the left foot with the left heel hitting the ground.

Photo #7: Gradually shift the weight to the left leg. Again, you are in **Bow Stance**: your left knee (the front knee) is mildly flexed with the right leg (the back leg) straight.

Photo #8: As the body weight is entirely shifted to the left leg, the right heel comes off the ground. You are ready to swing the right leg forward.

Photo #9: The right leg is swinging forward, and your right foot becomes parallel to the left foot (the front foot). The toes of the right foot (the back foot) gently touch the ground while the left foot continues to support the body. Now you are back in **Transitional Stance**.

Safety. The typical Tai Chi walk, the curved walk, has been replaced by natural walking or slowed natural walking in E Tai Chi. You always face forward without making turns, squatting, or kicking.

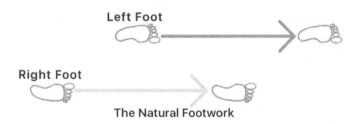

The footwork in natural walking and E Tai Chi.

Most postures in all the current Tai Chi styles involve a slow forward walking. The knee joint will sustain a lot of strain during walking forward because the position of the front knee is far away from the midline of the body. In contrast, the chance of getting knee injuries will be much lower during walking sideways or backward as the position of the knees is very close to the midline. Additionally, walking sideways requires much less flexion of the knee joints than walking forward. Because you walk sideways in most of the E Tai Chi postures, you can avoid over-flexion of the knees and maintain optimal knee-foot alignment. You may not feel pain when doing the sidestepping workout if you suffer from knee pain before practicing Tai Chi. Walking sideways not only poses a low risk of knee injuries but also offers some specific therapeutic potential (see below).

Since E Tai Chi involves only gentle hand/arm movements and regular standing or walking, it should not incur more risks than a person's usual daily activities do. When you practice the E Tai Chi sequences, you will slow down your walking pace. On the one hand, the slow execution of Tai Chi can provide a good workout on lower extremities and relax your mind. On the other hand, it may strain your knee joints if you are a beginner or at an advanced age. Therefore, I have designed **Transitional Stance** to solve this problem. Namely, you can take a break by placing your swinging foot parallel to the standing foot during the midswing phase of the gait cycle. See **Figure 2-1C**.

All these safety designs will minimize injuries induced by Tai Chi exercises. You can practice E Tai Chi safely anywhere, anytime, and in any position (sitting, standing, walking, or even lying). Thanks to its gentle arm/hand movements and regular standing or walking, E Tai Chi is safe, especially for older people.

Strength. In the E Tai Chi sequence, the majority of the postures involve sideways walking. E Tai Chi provides an efficient physical workout because walking sideways consumes over three times more energy than walking forward (Handford & Srinivasan, 2014). Older individuals have a reduced ability to take side steps to avoid obstacles (Gilchrist, 1998). They are at higher risk of falling laterally and suffering a hip fracture (Maki & McIlroy, 2006). Sideway training is used in rehabilitation in patients with stroke, brain injuries, or Parkinson's disease (Kim & Kim, 2014) (Bryant, Workman, Hou, Henson, & York, 2016). Therefore, sideways walking exercise will help prevent falls in older adults.

According to a recent study, the most common knee symptom among Tai Chi practitioners is lateral knee pain, which is consistent with iliotibial band syndrome (Yuan 苑, 2014). Strengthening exercises, including sidestepping, are an effective treatment for iliotibial band syndrome. Sidestep training has been used in physical therapy to alleviate back pain and pain disorders affecting lower extremities (ACE Physical Therapy and Sports Medicine Institute, 2015). Therefore, the emphasis on walking sideways in E Tai Chi not only decreases the risk of getting Tai Chi induced knee pain or injury but helps relieve knee pain due to other causes such as patellofemoral pain syndrome.

You can rise up onto tiptoes when practicing the advanced E Tai Chi. Standing or walking on your tiptoes can help improve balance, calf strength, posture, and ankle function.

E Tai Chi can be combined with a strength-training workout if you wear some weights on your wrists and ankles. You can make E Tai Chi an aerobic exercise by speeding up the hand/arm movements.

Serenity. E Tai Chi combines with Qigong, a specific Chinese breathing/meditation exercise like Yoga. You can easily coordinate your breathing with hand movements because all the hand/arm movements are symmetrical. E Tai Chi relaxes your body, reduces stress, promotes physical fitness, and cultivates the sensation of feeling good.

You can create your own E Tai Chi sequence by using the six basic hand movements and different ways of walking or standing. These hand /arm movements can be easily transformed further into any movements of existing Tai Chi styles. Therefore, E Tai Chi has laid a solid foundation for you if you wish to pursue traditional Tai Chi forms in the future.

The Study Plan for E Tai Chi

Level One E Tai Chi

Learn three hand/arm movements: Movements 1, 2, and 3. It takes maximum **10 minutes** to learn them.

Practice standing E Tai Chi with Movement 1, Movement 2, and Movement 3. It takes **five minutes** to master it.

Walk normally while performing Movements 1, 2, and 3. You can do it right away.

Learn the basic E Tai Chi sequence. You can practice it without hand/foot coordination instantly. It probably takes about **one to two hours** to master the hand/foot coordination.

In short, Level One E Tai Chi consists of Movements 1, 2, and 3 while standing and walking, and the basic E Tai Chi sequence.

Level Two E Tai Chi:

Perform Movements 1, 2, 3, 4, 5, and 6 while standing or walking, and practice the intermediate E Tai Chi sequence.

Level Three E Tai Chi:

Perform hand movements vertically and horizontally, pay attention to relaxation, and coordinate your breathing with hand/arm movements.

Therefore, you can master the Level One E Tai Chi within two to three hours. You can practice it for a few weeks before proceeding to learn Level Two or Level Three. If you can practice Level One E Tai Chi well and regularly, you will achieve most of the benefits of Tai Chi.

Keep in mind: Practice E Tai Chi with Five S's: Simplicity, Safety, Serenity, Strength, and Science.

Also, remember: Living your life with Five S's: Smile, Simplicity, Sympathy, Serenity, and Service. See my book: *Life and Medicine*.

In summary:

Level One E Tai Chi (two to three hours)
1. Movements 1, 2, and 3.
2. Perform while standing and walking.
3. Learn the basic sequence.

Level Two E Tai Chi (one to two days)
1. Movements 1 to 6.
2. Perform while standing and walking.
3. Learn the intermediate-level sequence.

Level Three E Tai Chi (You will reach the advanced level spontaneously after having become proficient in practicing Level Two E Tai Chi.)
1. All the above
2. The advanced level sequence.

Chapter 3. The Basics of E Tai Chi.

千里之行始于足下。
A journey of a thousand miles must begin with the first step.
—老子 (Lao Tzu, 571 B.C., Chinese Philosopher)

行路难

行路难，行路难。多歧路，今安在？
长风破浪会有时，直挂云帆济沧海！

Hard is the way, hard is the way.
Don't go astray! Whither today.
A time will come to ride the wind and cleave the waves,
I'll set my cloudlike sail to cross the sea which raves.
—李白 (Li Bai, 701－762, Chinese Poet)
Translated by 许渊冲 (Xu Yuanchong)

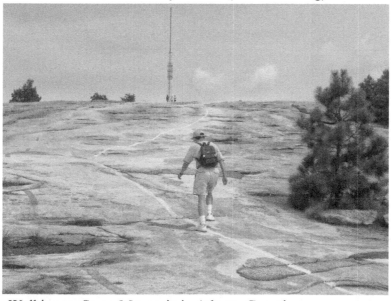

Walking up Stone Mountain in Atlanta, Georgia.

There are numerous hand/arm movements, stances, and kicks in traditional Tai Chi. For example, in his book about standardized Tai Chi, Professor Li Deyin (李德印教授) teaches 33 hand/arm movements, 10 stances, 14 ways of walking, and 6 types of kicking (Li 李, 2003). It scares away many potential Tai Chi learners.

In E Tai Chi, there are only five stances, three ways of walking, and six hand/arm movements without kicking, jumping, and squatting. You can turn your palms in any direction. You are doing it right if you do not feel awkward and can perform comfortably. After you have learned the basics in this chapter and the next chapter, you will go on to grasp E Tai Chi without difficulty and succeed in becoming a master of E Tai Chi.

Stances

There are many stances in traditional Tai Chi, including the Simplified 24-Form. Many of these different stances provide no proven health benefits and may even hurt your joints. There are only five simple stances in E Tai Chi as follows:

Stance One: **Normal Standing**.

Stance Two: **Routine Stance**.

Stance Three: **Transitional Stance**.

Stance Four: **Empty Stance**.

Stance Five: **Bow Stance**.

Stance One: Normal Standing

Stand naturally in a relaxed state with your feet shoulder-width apart and with knees straight. Feet are naturally placed with toes pointed forward. Keep your head upright and your eyes looking forward. Relax your shoulders. Hang your hands and arms loosely at your sides. See **Figure 3-1A**.

Almost all the Tai Chi books emphasize that the tip of the tongue should touch the roof of the mouth behind the upper teeth. It was believed that you could connect the imaginary "circulation" to let "qi (energy)" move around the body. You do not need to think about the position of your tongue in E Tai Chi. Anything natural and comfortable is fine.

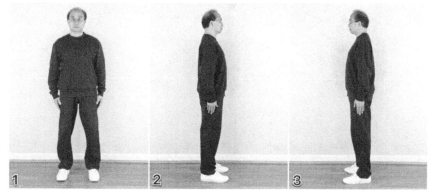

Figure 3-1A. Normal standing.

Stance Two: **Routine Stance**

Stand or move with the knees flexed at 10-20 degrees. Feet are naturally placed with toes pointed forward. See **Figure 3-1B**. When carrying out regular walking, you typically bend your knee joints to the same extent. If normal walking does not hurt you, then this angle of flexion will be appropriate. Use this stance most of the time when practicing E Tai Chi sequences.

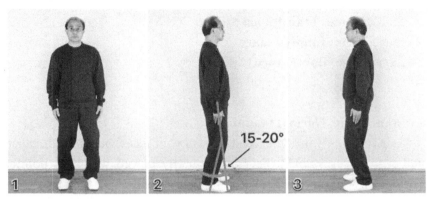

Figure 3-1B. Routine Stance.

The Important Point

Bend your knees to a lesser degree or do not flex them at all if you feel uncomfortable or pain in this stance.

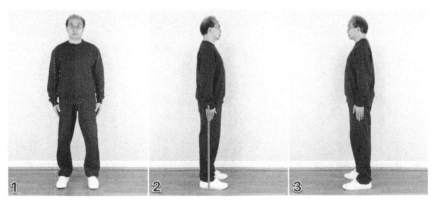

Figure 3-1Bb. Routine Stance without knee flexion (normal standing).

Stance Three: Transitional Stance

Stand with one foot (the right foot in the figure) supporting the body weight. Another foot (here the left foot) with the heel off the ground is placed parallel to the supporting foot. The toes of both feet are pointed forward. The knee (here the right knee) of the supporting leg is bent at 10-20 degrees. See **Figure 3-1C**. This stance is the typical posture in which we stand relaxedly when carrying on a casual conversation or waiting in line.

You can use this stance to do all the transitions from one posture to another posture when walking forward, backward, and sideways. This stance is unique and never seen in other styles of Tai Chi. It differs from the follow-up stance in Sun and Hao style Tai Chi. The back foot is positioned behind the front foot in Sun and Hao styles.

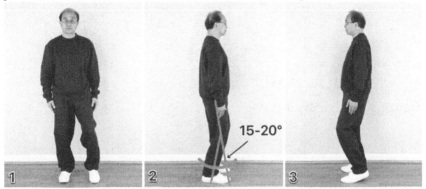

Figure 3-1C. Transitional Stance.

The Important Point. Bend your supporting knee to a lesser degree or do not flex it at all if you feel uncomfortable or pain in this stance.

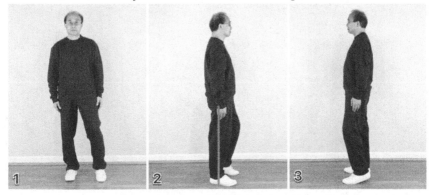

Figure 3-1Cc. Transitional Stance without rear knee flexion.

Stance Four: Empty Stance

Stand with the rear leg (the right leg in the figure) supporting the entire weight of the body. The back knee is flexed at 10-20 degrees. The toes of the front foot (here the left foot) are placed in the front and pointed forward, and the rear foot (here the right foot) is angled outward at 35-45 degrees. See **Figure 3-1D**. It happens only in Posture Five. See Posture Five in Chapter 6.

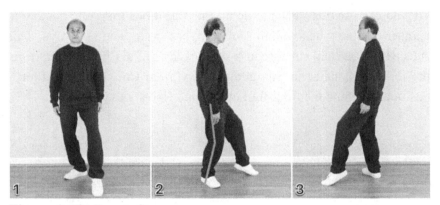

Figure 3-1D. Empty Stance.

The Important Point

Bend your rear knee to a lesser degree or do not flex it at all if you feel uncomfortable or pain in this stance.

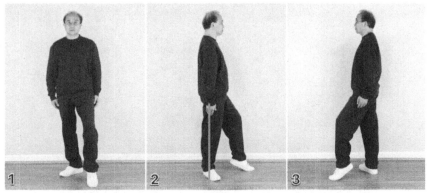

Figure 3-1Dd. Empty Stance without back knee flexion.

Stance Five: Bow Stance

If you walk forward slowly enough, you may find out that you adopt a bow stance that is seen in all styles of Tai Chi. Your front knee (the left knee in the figure) is mildly flexed with the front lower leg perpendicular to the ground and the back leg (here the right leg) straight. Your feet are shoulder-width apart with toes pointed forward. See **Figure 3-1E**. It is critical to perform this stance correctly. Otherwise, your knees will be damaged as I mentioned before. See the explanations in the walking section.

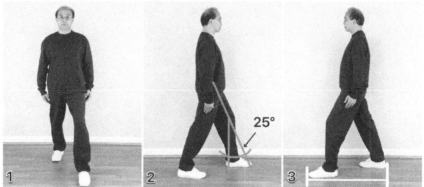

Figure 3-1E. Bow Stance.

The Important Point

Bend your front knee to a lesser degree and take shorter steps if you feel uncomfortable or pain in Bow Stance.

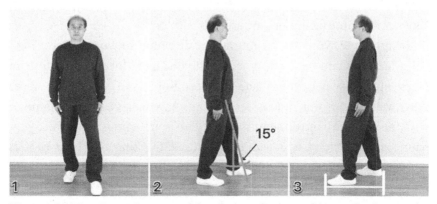

Figure 3-1Ee. Bow Stance with a lesser degree of knee flexion and a shorter step length.

Hands and Arms

Hands and Arms

Relax the hands with the fingers naturally positioned. Try to sink the shoulders and drop the elbows no matter what hand/arm movements you perform. This is one of the most important Tai Chi principles, which helps not only relax your body and mind but make your postures look elegant. You will feel relaxed and energetic if you follow this simple rule. This topic will be discussed in depth in the advanced E Tai Chi.

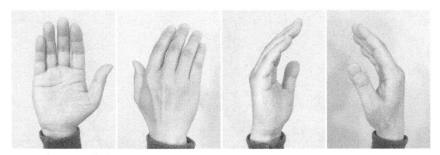

Figure 3-2A. Hands and fingers.

Direction of palms

Whether your palms face downward, upward, outward, inward, or in any direction does not matter too much as long as you feel comfortable and relaxed. Different styles of Tai Chi prefer various directions of the palms. No scientific evidence has shown that palm-facing-upward is superior or palm-facing-downward is healthier.

In principle, your palms follow the direction of your hands. Your palm faces toward the front if you push your hand forward. Your palm faces upward when your hand is ascending. And your palm faces downward when your hand is descending. As you have become familiar with the hand/arm movements in E Tai Chi, your actions will direct your palms automatically and naturally without thinking. Of course, it is much easier to obtain "qi" when you follow this rule. I will demonstrate the direction of palm movements in Movement 1 and Movement 2, which give rise to all the other hand/arm movements in E Tai Chi.

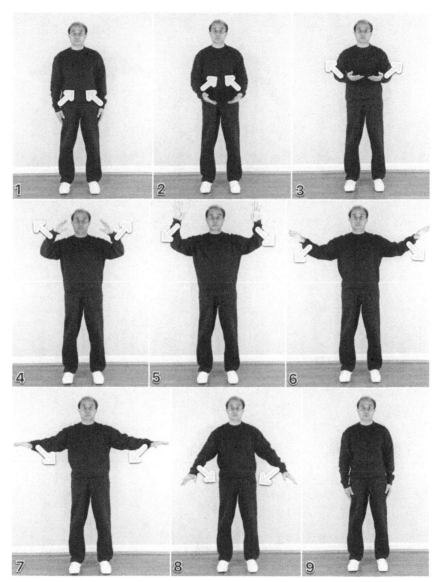

Figure 3-2B. Palm direction in Movement 1.

Key Points for **Figure 3-2B**.

Photo #1 to **Photo #3**. The palms face upward when the hands are ascending. **Photo #4**. Transition. The palms face inward. **Photo #5**. Transition. The palms face forward. **Photo #6** to **Photo #8**. The palms face downward when the hands are descending.

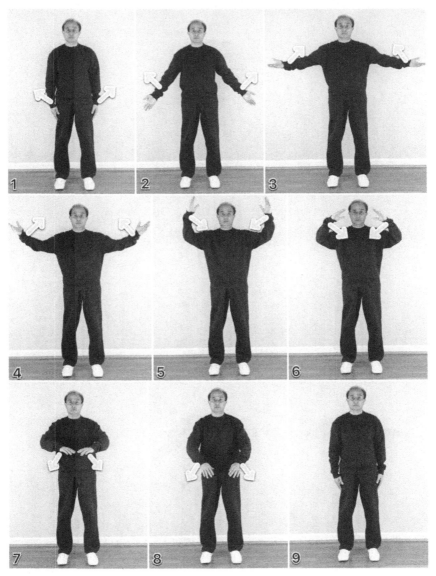

Figure 3-2C. Palm direction in Movement 2.

Key Points for **Figure 3-2C**.

Photo #1 to **Photo #3**. The palms face upward when the hands are ascending. **Photo #4**. Transition. The palms face inward. **Photo #5**. Transition. The palms face forward. **Photo #6** to **Photo #8**. The palms face downward when the hands are descending.

Hand and arm movements

They will be described in detail in Chapter 4.

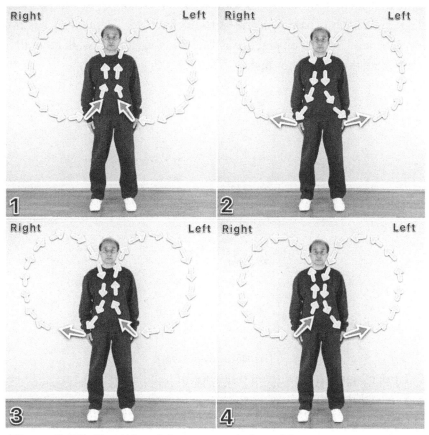

Figure 3-2D. Hand/Arm Movements 1, 2, and 3.

   Photo #1. Movement 1: simultaneously circle your left hand counterclockwise and right hand clockwise.

   Photo #2. Movement 2: simultaneously circle your left hand clockwise and right hand counterclockwise.

   Photo #3. Movement 3 (Leftward): simultaneously circle your left hand and right hand counterclockwise.

   Photo #4. Movement 3 (Rightward): simultaneously circle your left hand and right hand clockwise.

Walk

The typical traditional Tai Chi walk is a curved walk (see the diagram), which is hard to learn, not safe for older people, and has no health benefit. When you practice E Tai Chi, you can just walk naturally in any direction, slowly or fast.

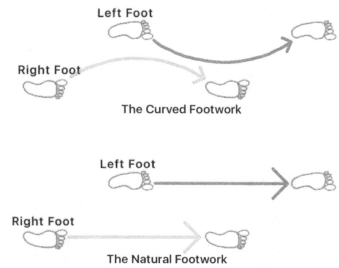

Upper Figure. The curved footwork in traditional Tai Chi.
Lower Figure. The footwork in natural walking and E Tai Chi.

Lift **the heel** up first and then the whole foot when you lift the foot to make a step. When performing slow walking in the E Tai Chi sequences, make sure not to over-flex the knee joint of the supporting leg. This principle applies to any walking (forward, backward, and sideward).

Walking forward: Walk forward naturally with **the heel** hitting the ground first. See **Figure 3-3A.**

Walking backward: Walk backward naturally with **the toes** touching the ground first. See **Figure 3-3B.**

Walking sideways: Walk naturally to one side with **the toes** contacting the ground first, and then the whole foot. See **Figure 3-3C.**

Walking Forward Naturally

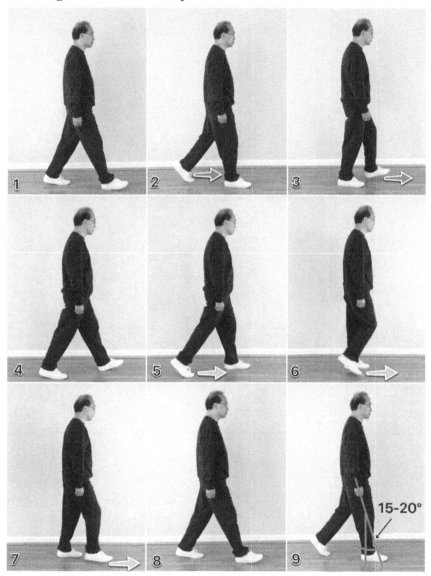

Figure 3-3A. Walking forward naturally.
Photo #1: Initial Contact. **Photo #2**: Loading Response. **Photo #3**: Midstance. **Photo #4**: Terminal Stance. **Photo #5**: Preswing. **Photo #6**: Initial Swing. **Photo #7**: Midswing. **Photo #8 (= Photo #1)**: Terminal Swing. **Photo #9**: The same as **Photo #2 (Loading Response)**. The peak flexion of the knee. See the key points for **Figure 3-3A** on Page 43.

Walking Backward Naturally

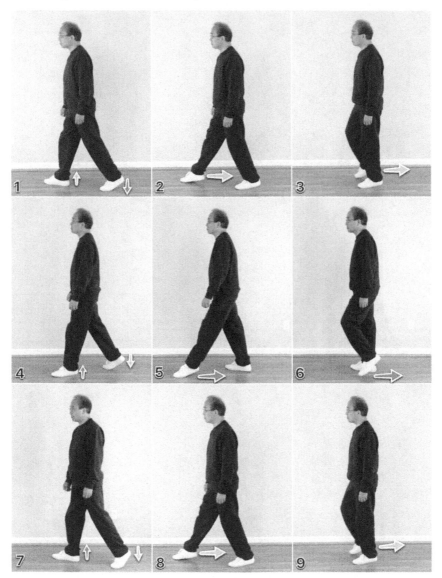

Figure 3-3B. Walking backward naturally.

Key points for **Figure 3-3B**.

Photo #1: The left foot is moving backward with the toes of the left foot touching the ground.

Photo #2: Shift the body weight to the left leg with the entire left foot contacting the ground. In the meantime, lift the right heel up and get ready to step back with the right foot.

(The left heel is naturally moved inward as the body weight is gradually shifted to the left leg. The inward movement of the heel should occur spontaneously because the resulting posture produces optimal body stability. The final posture is: the toes of the right foot, the front foot, are pointed forward, and the rear foot, the left foot, is angled outward at 35-45 degrees.)

Photo #3: The right foot is swinging backward. At this time, the right foot becomes parallel to the left foot.

Photo #4: The toes of the right foot touch the ground. Gradually shift the body weight to the right leg.

Photo #5: The body weight has moved entirely to the right leg. Lift the left heel up and get ready to step back with the left foot.

(The final posture is: the toes of the left foot (the front foot) are pointed forward, and the rear foot (the right foot) is angled outward at 35-45 degrees.)

Photo #6: The left foot is swinging backward and passing the right foot.

Photo #7(= Photo #1): The left foot continues to move backward and touches the ground with the toes of the left foot.

Photo #8 (= Photo #2): Shift your body weight to the left leg with the entire left foot contacting the ground. Lift the right heel up and get ready to step back with the right foot.

(The final posture is: the toes of the right foot (the front foot) are pointed forward, and the rear foot (the left foot) is angled outward at 35-45 degrees.)

Now you can repeat the same cycle of backward walking.

Photo #9= Photo #3.

Walking Sideways

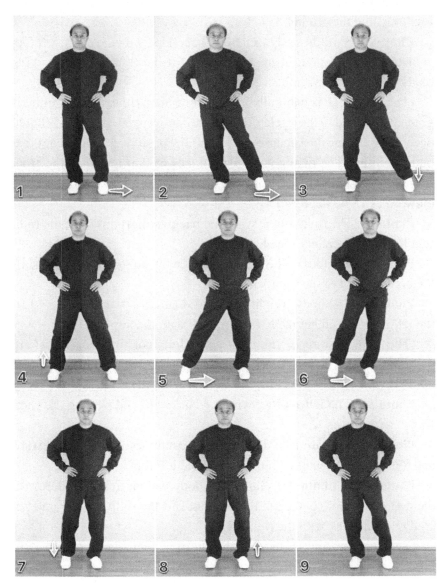

Figure 3-3C. Walking sideways.

Walk leftward. After you have shifted your weight to the right leg, take a step sideward left with your left foot. Lift the heel of the moving foot off the ground first and then the whole foot. The distance between your two feet is one to two feet wide. The toes of the left foot touch the ground first, and then the whole foot contacts the ground. The toes of the feet keep facing forward.

After your left foot has become in complete contact with the ground, gradually shift your body weight to the left leg. Then bring the right foot closer to the left foot and shift the weight back to the right leg. Repeat the same action if you continue to walk sideways left.

Walk rightward. Do it the same way with a different foot.

The above principle applies to all the sideward-moving postures (Postures One, Two, Three, Six, Seven, and Eight).

Key points for **Figure 3-3C**.

Photo #1: **Routine Stance** to **Transitional Stance**. Stand with feet shoulder-width apart. The knees are flexed at 10-20 degrees. Keep both feet pointed forward during walking sideways. Shift your body weight to the right leg. Lift the left heel up and get ready to step out.

Photo #2: Take a step sideways left with the left foot.

Photo #3: The toes of the left foot touch the ground.

Photo #4: Gradually shift the body weight to the left leg. At this moment, the weight is evenly distributed between both legs.

Photo #5: The body weight is fully shifted to the left leg with the right heel off the ground. You are ready to bring your right foot in.

Photo #6: Move the right foot toward the left foot.

Photo #7: The right foot comes in contact with the ground. The toes of the right foot touch the ground first. You are in **Transitional Stance** (the left leg is the supporting leg).

Photo #8: Gradually shift the body weight to the right leg. At this moment, the weight is evenly distributed between both legs. You are back to **Routine Stance**.

Photo #9: After having transferred all your weight back to the right leg, you are in **Transitional Stance** again (the right leg is the supporting leg). You are ready to take the second sideward step with the left foot.

If you want to walk sideways to the right, then you can start by taking a step sideways right with the right foot in the same way as described above.

Slow Walking in E Tai Chi Sequences

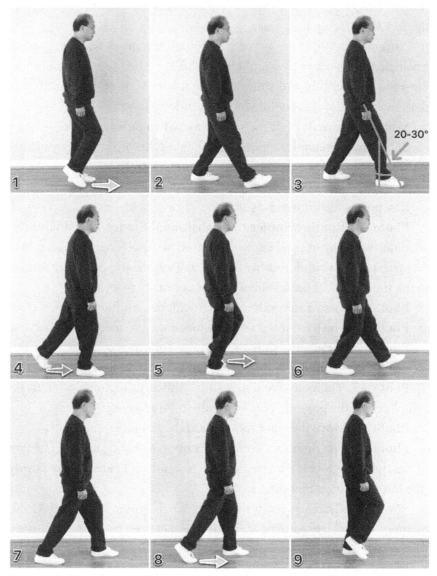

Figure 3-3D. Slow walking in E Tai Chi sequences.

Slow Walking in E Tai Chi Sequences

Keep the body upright. Lift **the heel** up first and then the whole foot when you lift the foot to make a step. This principle applies to any walking (forward, backward, and sideward).

Use the rear leg to push the body forward to shift the body weight to the front foot. This way will prevent the over-flexion of the supporting front leg. I propose that the flexion of the knees should not be over **20-30 degrees**, and the length of each step should be within **30 inches** (76 cm) in order to prevent knee injuries.

Key points for **Figure 3-3D**.

Photo #1: This is **Transitional Stance**: one of the legs (the left leg in the figure) is supporting the body weight while the toes of the other leg (here the right leg) gently touch the ground to maintain balance.

Photo #2: Step forward with the right foot. The right heel comes in contact with the ground.

Photo #3: Gradually shift the body weight to the right leg. Now, you are in **Bow Stance**: your front knee (here the right knee) is mildly flexed with the back leg (here the left leg) straight.

You should use the rear leg to push the body forward so that the front lower leg forms a 90-degree angle relative to the front foot or the ground. This is a standard **bow stance** in Chinese martial arts. When **you drive the body forward by the rear leg**, the front knee joint will not be over-flexed. This principle applies to all the forward movements.

Photo #4: As the body weight is fully shifted to the right leg, the left heel comes off the ground. You are ready to swing the left leg forward.

Photo #5: The left leg swings forward until it becomes parallel to the right leg. The toes of the left foot gently touch the ground. Now you are back in **Transitional Stance**.

Photo #6: Step forward with the left foot with the left heel hitting the ground.

Photo #7: Gradually shift the weight to the left leg. Again, you are in **Bow Stance**: your left knee (the front knee) is mildly flexed with the right leg (the back leg) straight.

Photo #8: As the body weight is fully shifted to the left leg, the right heel comes off the ground. You are ready to swing the right leg forward.

Photo #9: The right leg is swinging forward, and your right foot becomes parallel to the left foot (the front foot). The toes of the right foot (the back foot) gently touch the ground while the left foot continues to support the body. Now you are back in **Transitional Stance**.

Breathing

You should breathe spontaneously and naturally in the beginning. As you become familiar with the E Tai Chi movements, you can coordinate your breathing with your hand movements.

Traditional Tai Chi styles were not designed according to the rhythm of breath. Therefore, if emphasizing breathing synchronization when performing traditional Tai Chi, one has to carry out coordinated breathing and natural breathing alternately. The process is complicated to learn. Since E Tai Chi consists of only symmetrical hand movements, you can synchronize your breathing with the hand movements from the beginning to the end easily and comfortably.

In principle, breathe in when circling your arms up, and breathe out when circling your arms down. If you are performing alternate movements (Movement 4, 5, and 6), choose one of the arms as an indicator for breathing pattern, e.g., the left arm/hand.

There is no need to do so-called reverse abdominal breathing, which is not practical, especially for older or overweight people. The breathing method in E Tai Chi will be discussed in depth in the complete book. Just breathe naturally and comfortably at this time.

Key Points for **Figure 3-4**.

Photo#1 to **Photo#4**. Movement 1. Breathe in when the hands are going up. Breathe out when the hands are going down.

Photo#5 to **Photo#8**. Movement 2. Breathe in when the hands are going up. Breathe out when the hands are going down.

Photo#9 to **Photo #12**. Movement 3 (Leftward). Breathe in when the hands are going up. Breathe out when the hands are going down.

Photo#13 to **Photo#16**. Movement 3 (Rightward). Breathe in when the hands are going up. Breathe out when the hands are going down.

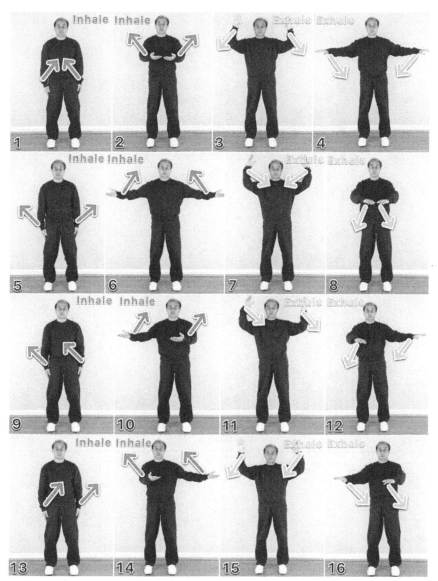

Figure 3-4. Breathing coordinated with the hand/arm movements.

Chapter 4. Hand/Arm Movements

早发白帝城
朝辞白帝彩云间，千里江陵一日还。
两岸猿声啼不住，轻舟已过万重山。

LEAVING THE WHITE KING'S TOWN AT DAWN
Leaving at dawn the White King crowned with rainbow cloud,
I have sailed a thousand miles through Three Georges in a day.
With monkeys' sad adieus the riverbanks are loud;
My boat has left ten thousand mountains far away.

—李白 (Li Bai, 701－762, Chinese Poet)
Translated by 许渊冲 (Xu Yuanchong)

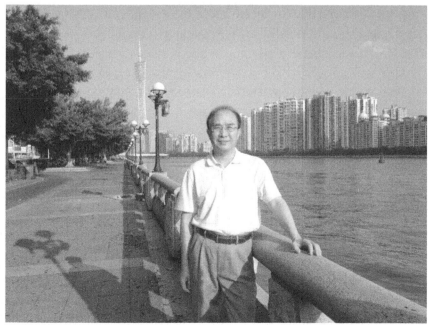

Walking along the north bank of the Pearl River in Guangzhou, China.

All the Tai Chi movements can be condensed to one circular hand movement. Therefore, E Tai Chi requires only **one** basic hand movement: circle your hands in front of your body. However, you will have a total of six different hand movements when you circle your hands simultaneously, sequentially, clockwise, or counterclockwise.

In this book, I circle my left hand and right hand on the left and right sides of my body, respectively, in order to clearly demonstrate the six hand movements and facilitate the learning process. However, when you perform the circular hand/arm movements, your hands or arms can be overlapped (crossed over the midline of your body) as long as you feel good. What you feel comfortable is right. Again, there is no strict rule in E Tai Chi. E Tai Chi is for your personal health only, not for fighting or competition. As a matter of fact, these six hand movements include all the fighting techniques in traditional Tai Chi.

Usually, you perform these circular hand movements vertically in front of your body because most of the typical Tai Chi hand movements are executed this way. Therefore, I focus on demonstrating vertical hand movements. However, you can play them diagonally, horizontally, or in any direction you like. In the advanced E Tai Chi, you perform the hand movements both vertically and horizontally. You will be surprised that Tai Chi can be practiced this way or any way you want.

As mentioned previously, whether your palms face downward, upward, outward, inward, or in any direction does not matter too much if you feel comfortable and relaxed. Different styles of Tai Chi prefer various directions of the palms. No scientific evidence shows that palm-facing-up is superior, or the palm-facing-down is healthier.

In principle, your palms follow the direction of your hands. Your palm faces toward the front if you push your hand forward. The palm faces upward when the hand is ascending. And the palm faces downward when the hand is descending. It is much easier to obtain "qi" when you follow this rule. The concept of "qi" (energy?) will be discussed in the science book.

The distance between your face/chest and your hands is usually about 1 foot (30 cm). However, you can use any range you want.

There are only six hand movements in E Tai Chi. It's simple, right? One of these movements (Movement 4) is **Cloud Hands (Wave Hands like Clouds)**, which exists in all styles of Tai Chi and is executed in a similar way: circle your hands sequentially in front of your torso. Principally, all the Tai Chi movements should look like floating clouds if you can perform them well. I would call Movement 4 "**Standard Cloud Hands**."

Nowadays, "cloud" is a hot name. We have cloud computing, cloud storage, and cloud-based anything. Therefore, I call the remaining five movements "Cloud Hands" too, but with some modifiers. I can guarantee that these five movements are entirely brand new, and no one has practiced them this way before. For example, all Tai Chi practitioners move their hands vertically to perform Standard Cloud Hands. Why can't we circle our hands horizontally, obliquely, or in the reverse direction? What Tai Chi masters did or what Tai Chi teachers taught is not the only way one can practice Tai Chi well and creatively. This is the reason that there are so many Tai Chi styles.

However, only in E Tai Chi, you can practice Tai Chi creatively. **The rule is "no rule" in E Tai Chi.** After you have learned the basics, you can practice E Tai Chi any way you desire. You can design E Tai Chi sequences by yourself. No one will say that you are performing E Tai Chi the wrong way. Again, E Tai Chi means simple, safe, and gentle.

The six E Tai Chi hand movements are named as follows:

Movement 1: Ascending Cloud Hands,
Movement 2: Descending Cloud Hands,
Movement 3: Concurrent Cloud Hands,
Movement 4: Standard Cloud Hands,
Movement 5: Reverse Cloud Hands,
Movement 6: Bidirectional Cloud Hands.

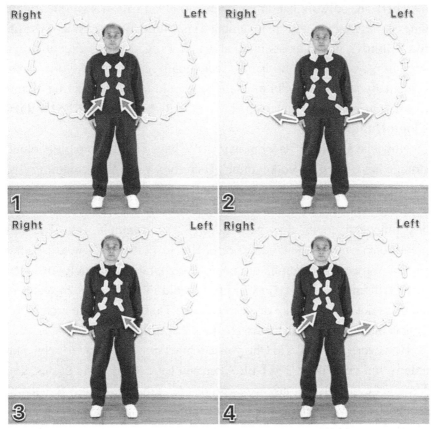

Figure 4-0. The motions of Movements 1, 2, and 3. The arrows show the direction of hand movements. The large arrows indicate the starting points of hand movements.

Photo #1. Movement 1: simultaneously circle your hands up through the midline of the body and circle your hands down and out to your sides (simultaneously circle your left hand counterclockwise and your right hand clockwise).

Photo #2. Movement 2: simultaneously circle your hands up, out to your sides, and circle your hands down along the midline of the body (simultaneously circle your left hand clockwise and your right hand counterclockwise).

Photos #3 and **#4. Movement 3**: simultaneously circle your hands in the same direction (counterclockwise or clockwise) in front of the body.

76

If you simultaneously circle your hands up through the midline of the body (the left-hand circles counterclockwise and the right hand clockwise), you are doing **Movement 1**, which I name "**Ascending Cloud Hands.**" See **Photo #1** in **Figure 4-0**.

If you simultaneously circle your hands up to your sides (the left hand circles clockwise and the right-hand counterclockwise), you are doing **Movement 2**, which I call "**Descending Cloud Hands.**" See **Photo #2** in **Figure 4-0**.

When you simultaneously circle your hands to the left or to the right (both hands circle counterclockwise or clockwise), you are performing **Movement 3,** which I name "**Concurrent Cloud Hands.**" See **Photo #3** and **Photo#4** in **Figure 4-0**.

Movements 4 to 6 will be described in detail in the complete book of E Tai Chi.

Movements 1, 2, and 3 are so simple that you can learn how to do them within minutes. If you do not want to go further, you can practice standing or walking E Tai Chi right away. That means you perform Movements 1, 2, and 3 while walking regularly.

Furthermore, you can master the basic E Tai Chi sequence within an hour. You can tell your friends and family members that you know how to practice Tai Chi and enjoy it. (See Chapter 6: Basic E Tai Chi Sequence.)

Because you can learn and enjoy E Tai Chi with minutes or hours, you will have the confidence to continue to learn more and avoid the failure many Tai Chi learners have suffered due to the awkward beginning movements in all the Tai Chi styles.

If you can practice the standing or walking E Tai Chi, and the basic E Tai Chi sequence every day for 20-30 minutes, you will achieve almost all the health benefits of Tai Chi.

Of course, performing the somewhat complicated movements like Movements 4, 5, and 6 will build up your confidence and make you enjoy more the beauty of Tai Chi. Even though Movements 4, 5, and 6 appear complicated, you can learn them within 1-2 hours. The fluidity of the movements, the relaxation of the body, and coordination of leg/arm movements can be gradually mastered as you practice E Tai Chi regularly.

Movement 1: Ascending Cloud Hands

Let us start to practice it. Simultaneously raise both hands up in front of your torso slowly and comfortably. Your hands move upward in a circular manner toward the midline. After your hands meet at upper abdomen or chest level, spread your hands out and raise them overhead or to any height you like. Then, move your hands circularly downward and outward, and gently drop them back to your sides.

In other words, you simultaneously circle your right hand clockwise and your left hand counterclockwise in front of your body. It does not matter how close or far your hands/arms are away from your body if you feel comfortable. Similarly, you do not need to worry about how high your hands will ascend although the most natural and comfortable height of your hands is at the level of your head or slightly overhead.

In principle, your palms follow the direction of your hands. Your palm faces toward the front if you push your hand forward. The palm faces upward when the hand is ascending and faces downward when the hand is descending. The distance between your face/chest and your hands is usually about 1 foot (30 cm). However, you do not have to think about the direction of the palms at all in the beginning. Do whatever you feel comfortable. You are done with the first movement, Movement 1.

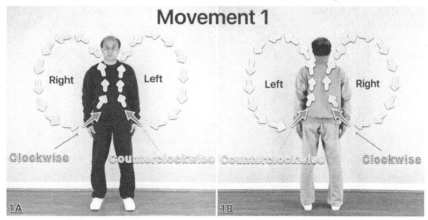

Photo 1A and **1B**. Movement 1: simultaneously circle your left hand counterclockwise and your right hand clockwise. The large red arrows indicate the starting points of hand movements.

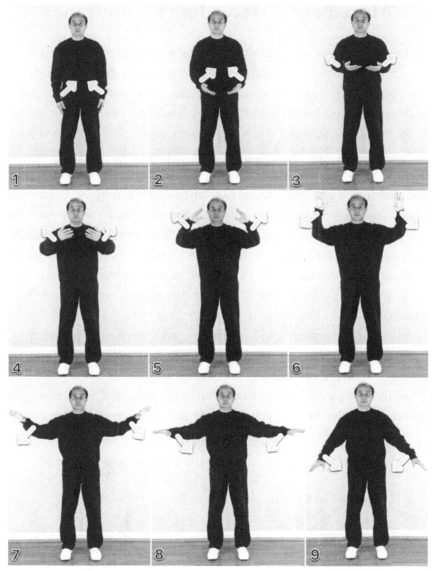

Figure 2-1. Movement 1 performed vertically. The arrows show the direction of hand movements.

Key points for **Figure 4-1**.

Photo #1: Normal Standing. Stand with feet shoulder-width apart. Your hands rest at your sides. The knees are straight. Keep your torso upright. This is the starting stance for the following actions.

Photo #2: Circle your hands up through the midline of your body. The palms are directed upward when the hands are ascending. The fingers of both hands point to each other diagonally. You look like you are holding a big ball in front of your body.

Photo #3: The hands continue to ascend. They are at shoulder level at this moment.

Photo #4: When your hands are raised above the chest, your palms gradually turn (pronate) and face backward.

Photo #5: The palms are directed to face inwards during the transition from facing upward to facing forward.

Photo #6: When the hands are lifted above the head, the palms turn to face forward. You look like you are pushing the ball away.

Photo #7: The palms face downward while the hands are descending to your sides. However, you do not have to think about the direction of the palms at all in the beginning. Do whatever you feel comfortable.

Photo #8: The hands continue to descend. They are at shoulder level at this moment.

Photo #9: The hands are returning to your sides.

Movement 2: Descending Cloud Hands

This movement is almost the same as Movement 1 except moving in the opposite direction.

Simultaneously spread and raise your arms to the sides in a circular manner outwardly and upwardly. At chest level, your hands move circularly up and toward the midline until they are lifted above the head. Then, your hands start to go inward and downward in front of the torso. Finally, your hands gently drop back to your sides.

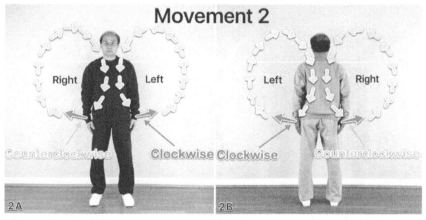

Photos 2A and **2B**. Movement 2: Simultaneously circle your left hand clockwise and your right hand counterclockwise. The large red arrows indicate the starting points of hand movements.

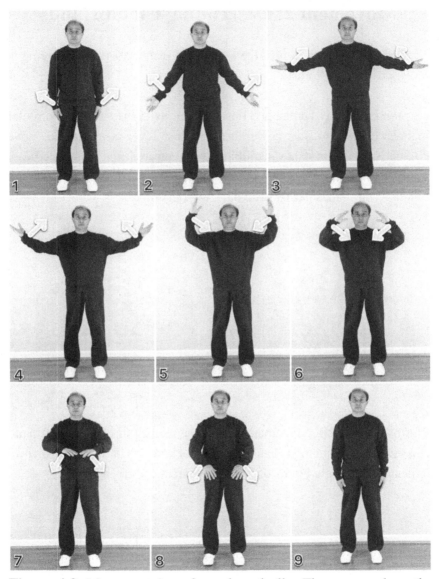

Figure 4-2. Movement 2 performed vertically. The arrows show the direction of hand movements.

Key points for **Figure 4-2**

Photo #1: **Normal Standing**. Stand naturally with feet shoulder-width apart.

Photo #2: Your hands are circling up to the sides. As the arms rotate out, the palms gradually turn and face forward.

Photo #3: The hands continue to ascend with the palms facing upward. The hands are at shoulder level at this moment.

Photo #4: The palms face inward as the hands are raised above shoulder level.

Photo #5: When the hands are raised overhead, the palms turn to face forward. Hereafter, the hands start to descend through the midline of the body.

Photo #6: The hands continue to incline through the midline with the palms facing downward.

Photo #7: The hands are at shoulder level.

Photo #8: The hands are returning to your sides.

Photo #9: Your hands have returned to your sides. You are back to **Normal Standing**.

Movement 3: Concurrent Cloud Hands

Circle both arms vertically in front of your body continuously. In other words, both hands move together in the same direction, clockwise or counterclockwise.

If your hands move circularly toward the left, then you realized you are practicing Movement 1 with your left arm and Movement 2 with your right arm. Similarly, if your hands move circularly toward the right, then you are practicing Movement 1 with your right arm and Movement 2 with your left arm. Namely, simultaneously practicing Movement 1 and Movement 2 with different hands is equal to practicing Movement 3.

Movement 1 + Movement 2 = Movement 3.

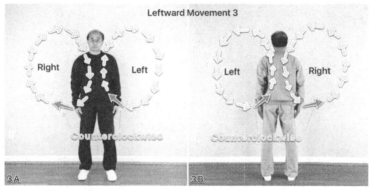

Photos 3A and **3B**. Movement 3 (Leftward): Simultaneously circle your left hand and right hand counterclockwise.

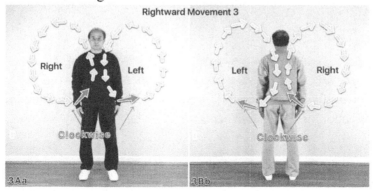

Photos 3Aa and **3Bb**. Movement 3 (Rightward): Simultaneously circle your left hand and right hand clockwise.

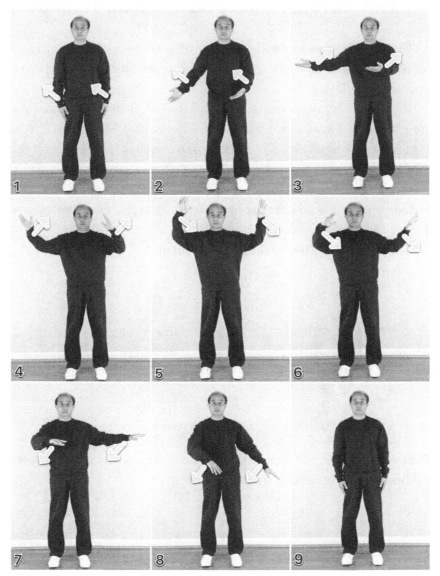

Figure 4-3A. Leftward Movement 3 performed vertically. The arrows show the direction of hand movements.

Key points for **Figure 4-3A**

Leftward Movement 3. Both hands simultaneously circle counterclockwise in front of the body.

Photo #1: **Normal Standing**. Stand naturally with feet shoulder-width apart.

Photo #2: Your right hand circles up to the side while your left hand circles up through the midline of the body.

Photo #3: The hands continue to ascend with the palms facing upward.

Photo #4: The palms face inward as the hands raised above shoulder level.

Photo #5: The hands have raised above the head with the palms facing forward. Hereafter, the right hand starts to descend through the midline while the left hand moves down to the side.

Photo #6: The hands continue to incline with the palms facing downward.

Photo #7: The hands are at shoulder level.

Photo #8: The hands are returning to your sides.

Photo #9: Your hands have returned to your sides. You are back to **Normal Standing**.

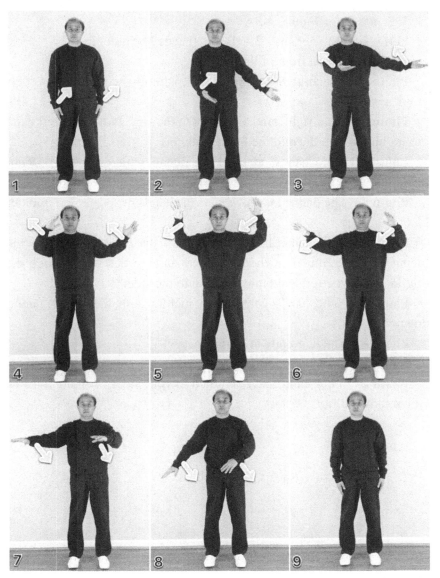

Figure 4-3B. Rightward Movement 3 performed vertically. The arrows show the direction of hand movements

Chapter 5. Practice E Tai Chi while Standing or Walking

Worry only about the things that are in your control, the things that can be influenced and changed by your actions, not about the things that are beyond your capacity to direct or alter.

—M. A. Soupios and Panos Mourdoukoutas
(Authors of *The Ten Golden Rules: Ancient Wisdom from the Greek Philosophers on Living the Good Life*) (Mourdoukoutas, 2012)

As mentioned above, you can practice E Tai Chi anywhere, in the park, in the office, in the backyard, in the living room, and even in the bathroom.

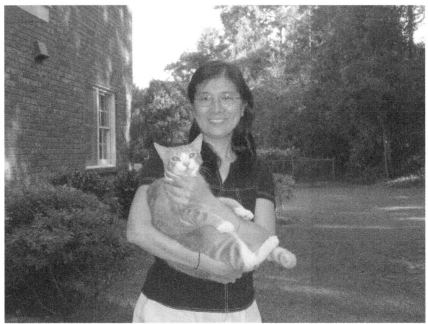

In loving memory of our cat, Bobo.

E Tai Chi while Standing

Routine Stance

Stand naturally in a relaxed state with feet shoulder-width apart. Your hands and arms hang loosely at your sides. Bend your knees to 10-20-degrees. Please make sure not to flex your knees too much because over-flexion can injury your knee joints. Keep your eyes looking straight ahead and breathe naturally and peacefully. Then, you are ready to practice the hand/arm movements of E Tai Chi (please refer to the previous chapter), and coordinate hand movements with your torso and leg movements.

The Important Point

Bend your knees to a lesser degree or do not flex your knees at all if you feel uncomfortable or pain in Routine Stance or Transitional Stance.

Practice Standing Movement 1

Standing in the way described above, start to practice Movement 1 (please refer to the previous chapter for the detailed description of Movement 1). As you slowly raise your arms, slowly straighten your knee joints. When your hands descend, your torso will sink with gentle flexion of your knees and return to the starting posture. Then you can repeat the same movement as many times as you like, usually 5-10 times. You look like you are swimming breaststroke. See **Figure 5-1A**.

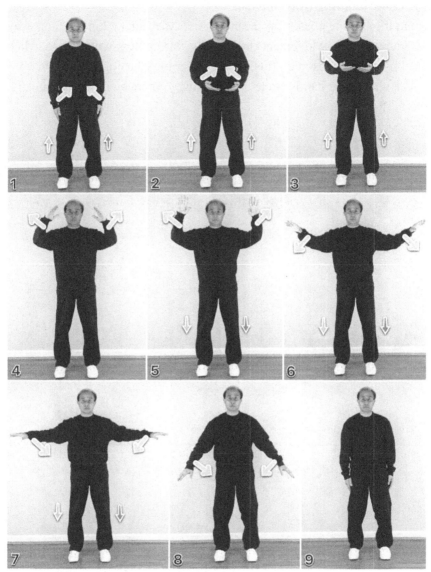

Figure 5-1A. Perform Movement 1 while standing.

Practice Standing Movement 2

In the starting posture, you can practice Movement 2 in the same way as you perform Movement 1. Namely, straighten your knees when circling your hands and arms up. Gently sink your torso and flex your knees when your hands circle down. Now, you are swimming butterfly. Do 5-10 repetitions.

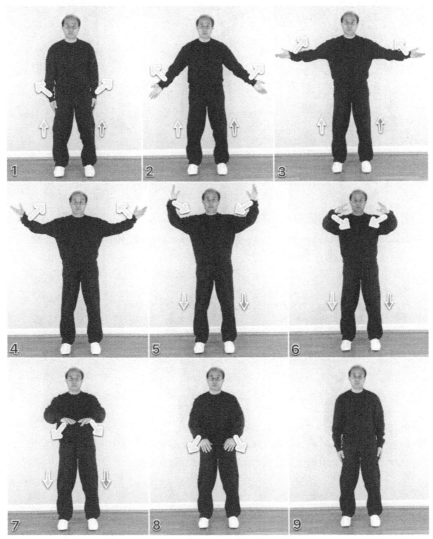

Figure 5-1B. Perform Movement 2 while standing.

Practice Standing Movement 3

In Routine Stance, you can practice Movement 3 in the same way as you perform standing Movements 1 and 2. Namely, straighten your knees when circling your hands and arms up. Gently sink your torso and flex your knees when circling your hands down. Then you return to the original posture and repeat the same movement again. Do 5-10 repetitions.

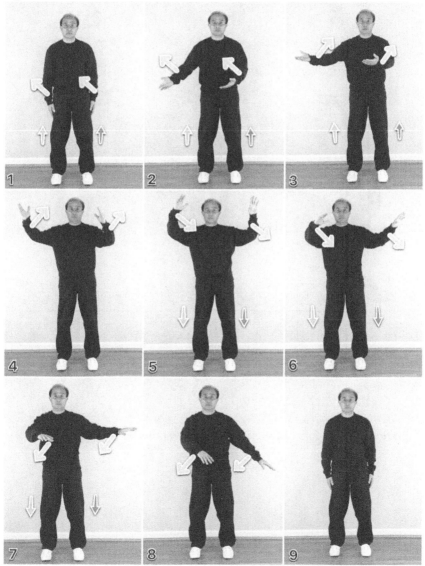

Figure 5-1C. Perform Movement 3 while standing (leftward).

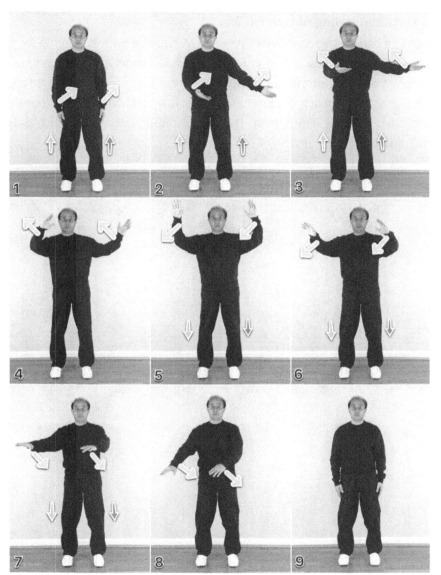

Figure 5-1D. Perform Movement 3 while standing (rightward).

E Tai Chi while Walking Forwards (E Tai Chi Walk)

Normal walking is undoubtedly one of the best physical exercises for everybody, especially for senior citizens. The shortcoming of regular walking is a lack of hand/arm exercises. E Tai Chi walking is the combination of Tai Chi hand movements and a regular walk. Through E Tai Chi, you can achieve the health benefits of both walking and Tai Chi. When doing E Tai Chi walking in an open space, you can breathe the fresh air and enjoy the beauty of Tai Chi fluidity.

It should be straightforward that you practice the above six hand movements while you take a natural walk. No precise hand-leg coordination is required. Just walk normally while performing the hand movements of E Tai Chi. You can walk circularly in a park, in your living room, in your yard, or in your office.

Practicing walking E Tai Chi is like swimming on land. Think about it, you are swimming breaststroke when doing Movement 1; you are swimming butterfly when doing Movement 2; swimming backstroke when doing Movement 4; and doing the crawl when practicing Movement 5.

You may be surprised that people will come up to you and ask, "What're you doing with these movements?" You can tell them you are practicing E Tai Chi and can be their teacher.

Generally, start with Movement 1 and end with Movement 6. Nevertheless, you can perform them in any sequence or just play some of them. Again, E Tai Chi has no strict standards. You are doing the right thing when you feel safe and comfortable.

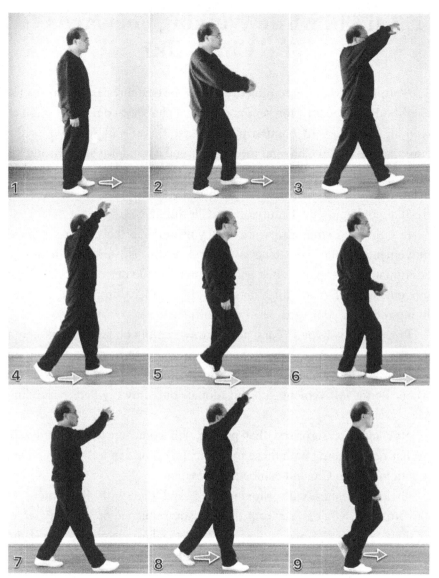

Figure 5-2A. Walking normally and performing Movement 1.

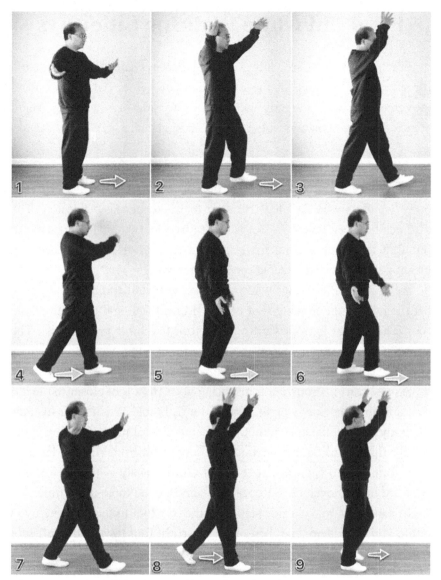

Figure 5-2B. Walking normally and performing Movement 3.

E Tai Chi while Walking Sideways

Practicing E Tai Chi while walking sideways is especially suitable for exercising indoors, in the office, and at home. All the six hand movements can be perfectly incorporated to sideways walking. There are six sideward postures in the E Tai Chi sequence.

As you start to circle both hands or the leading hand up, make a side step left with your left foot and, at the same time, gradually shift your body weight to the left leg. Be sure to make an easy sidestep. The distance between your two feet is one to two feet wide. The toes of the left foot touch the ground first, and then the whole foot contacts the ground. The toes of the feet keep facing forward.

As in regular sideways walking, when you start to take a side step, lift the heel of the moving foot off the ground first and then the whole foot. The toes of the sideward-moving foot touch the ground first. The above principle applies to all the sideward-moving postures (Postures One, Two, Three, Six, Seven, and Eight).

As you start to drop your arms, bring your right foot closer to the left foot and shift the bodyweight back to the right leg. When a leg sustains the body weight, the knee joint on the same side of the leg will be in the mildly flexed position. Your body weight shifts from right to left and then from left to right alternately and continuously while performing leftward hand movements. Repeat the same action three more times.

In summary, make a side step with the left foot to the left when you circle your hands up, and then move the right foot toward the left foot as your hands are descending.

After you have finished the last leftward hand movement, walk sideways rightward back to the starting location in the same way as you do in the leftward walking.

In other words, when you circle your hands up, take a step out rightward with your right foot and gradually shift your weight to the right leg. When your hands are going down, move the left foot closer to the right foot and gradually shift the weight back to the left leg. Repeat the same movements four times until you return to the starting location.

In the beginning, you may simply walk sideways while performing hand movements without any coordination. As you have become familiar with hand/foot movements, you will coordinate your hands and feet automatically. As I said before, any coordination is fine if you feel good. There are no absolute rules.

In principle, as your leading hand circles up, take a step out sideward with the leading leg; as your leading hand circles down, take a step sideward with the trailing leg.

How to perform E Tai Chi movements while walking sideways will be described in depth in Chapter 6.

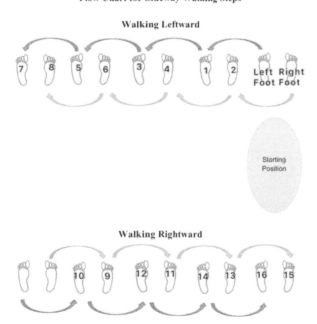

Flow Chart for Sideway Walking Steps

Walking Leftward

Walking Rightward

See details in the E Tai Chi sequence.

Sideward Movement 1 (Posture One in the basic E Tai Chi sequence)

Sideward Movement 2 (Posture Two in the basic E Tai Chi sequence)

Sideward Movement 3 (Posture Three in the basic E Tai Chi sequence)

E Tai Chi while Walking Backwards

As described above, you can perform all the Movements 1 to 6 comfortably when you walk forward and sideways. However, it is more natural to walk backward while playing only Movement 2, Movement 3, or Movement 5.

The safest way to practice walking backward is to walk slowly in a straight sidewalk, in a gym, or in a living room. Try not to coordinate your steps with hand movements at this stage. Just walk backward naturally and perform Movement 2, Movement 3, or Movement 5 at the same time. You will learn the hand-foot coordination when studying the E Tai Chi sequences later.

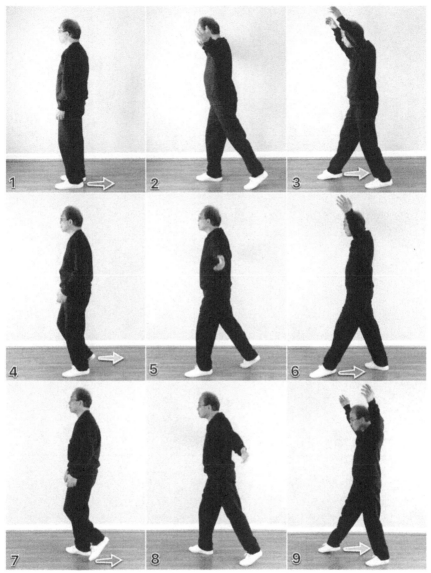

Figure 5-4A. Perform Movement 2 while walking backward naturally.

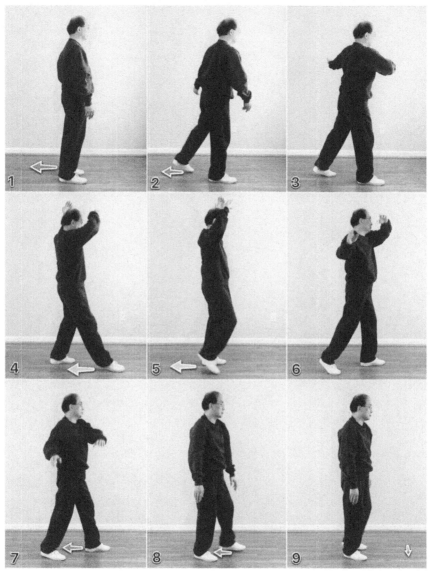

Figure 5-4B. Perform Movement 3 while walking backward naturally.

E Tai Chi while Marching in Space

You can do this exercise anywhere, inside or outside your house and your office. You can even watch TV news in the morning while performing E Tai Chi at the same time.

Initially, you do not need to coordinate your steps with your hand movements. As you get familiar with all the hand movements, you can quickly achieve the hand and foot coordination.

Principally, raise one of your feet when you circle your hands (or one of your hands) up and drop the foot back to the ground when circling your hands down. Do 5-10 repetitions with each foot.

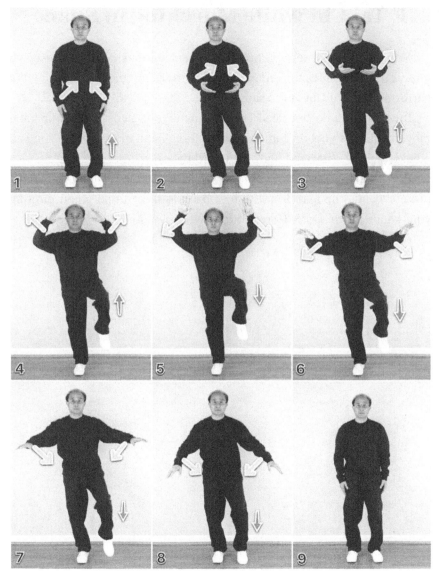

Figure 5-5A. March in space while performing Movement 1

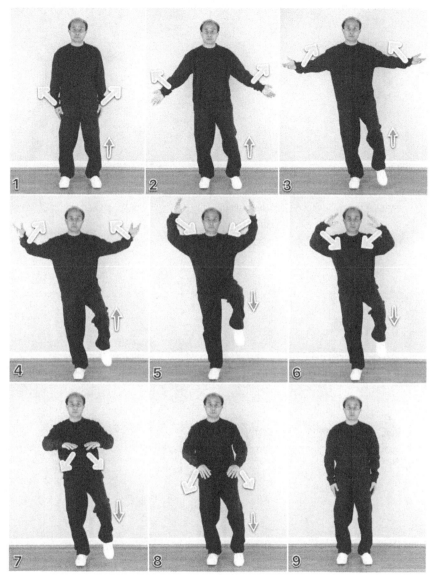

Figure 5-5B. March in space while performing Movement 2.

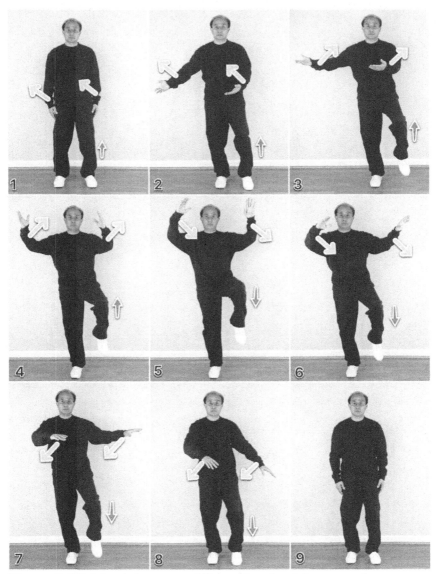

Figure 5-5C. March in space while performing Movement 3.

E Tai Chi with Weights

One of the shortcomings of traditional Tai Chi is a lack of upper body and aerobic exercises.

You can build up your upper body/arm strength by holding dumbbells or any weights while performing E Tai Chi. Especially, Movements 1, 2, 3, 4, and 5 can be perfectly integrated into weight exercises. How much weight you want to use is up to you. I suppose 1 to 2 pounds would be a good choice for walking and 2-5 pounds for standing. Please see the demonstrations (**Figure 5-6A** and **Figure 5-6B**). I practice E Tai Chi with 1.5-pound (0.68 kg) wrist weights, which I bought at Wal-Mart for $8.95.

Furthermore, you can wear weights on your ankles if you want to strengthen your leg muscles. I do not recommend ankle weights for walking due to safety reasons. It would be safe to wear ankle weights when standing or marching in space. You are still able to maintain the smoothness and relaxation of Tai Chi with weights on your wrists and ankles.

You can turn E Tai Chi into aerobic exercises if you perform the circular hand/arm movements fast with some weights on your wrists and ankles. You can even run in space while doing E Tai Chi Movements 4 and 5. However, you should consult your medical doctor first before starting an aerobic exercise.

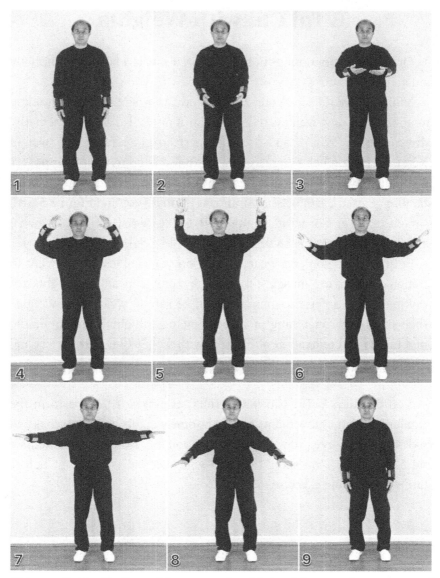

Figure 5-6A. Perform Movement 1 with weights on the wrists and practice standing on tiptoe (see Photos 4, 5, and 6).

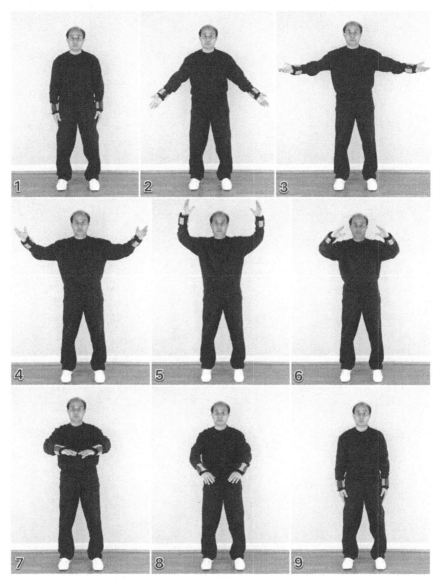

Figure 5-6B. Perform Movement 2 with weights on the wrists and practice standing on tiptoe (see Photos 4, 5, and 6).

Chapter 6. The Basic E Tai Chi Sequence

元夕

蛾儿雪柳黄金缕，笑语盈盈暗香去。

众里寻他千百度，蓦然回首，那人却在，灯火阑珊处。

The Lantern Festival Night

In gold-thread dress, with moth or willow ornaments,

Giggling, she melts into the throng with trails of scents.

But in the crowd once and again

I look for her in vain.

When all at once I turn my head,

I find her there where lantern light is dimly shed

—辛弃疾 (Xin Qiji, 1140 - 1207, Chinese Poet)

Translated by 许渊冲 (Xu Yuanchong)

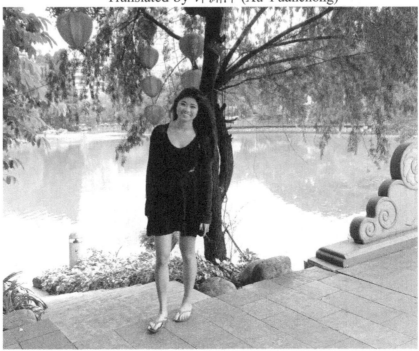

Megan, my daughter, standing under the lanterns in China.

The above poem tells the truth when it comes to Tai Chi learning. All of a sudden, you may find out that **E Tai Chi** is just right here and is so easy to learn after finishing reading this chapter.

It will be very easy for you to master the basic E Tai Chi sequence after you have learned the standing and walking E Tai Chi postures, as described in Chapter 5. Here, you just practice a series of hand/arm movements (from Movement 1 to Movement 3) while standing or walking. However, you will slow down your walking rhythm and emphasize the coordination of hand and foot movements. In the beginning, you can practice the sequence without any coordination.

I designed the walking sequence of E Tai Chi with reference to various styles of Tai Chi. Walk four steps sideways to the left and return to the original place. Then, walk four steps forward and walk four steps back to the starting location. However, you can take as many steps as you like. Also, you can walk sideward to the right side instead of walking leftward. All actions are symmetrical.

You can wear weights on your wrists if you wish to intensify muscular training. You are still able to maintain the smoothness and relaxation of Tai Chi with weights.

The basic sequence consists of five postures plus Starting Posture and Closing Posture. They are summarized as follows:

Simplified Flow Chart for the Basic E Tai Chi Sequence

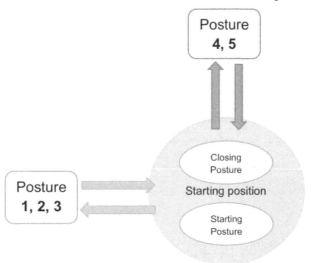

These postures are easy to remember.

Perform Movements **1** and **2** while standing in **Starting** and **Closing Postures,** respectively.

Perform Movements **1, 2,** and **3** while walking sideways in **Postures One, Two,** and **Three,** respectively.

Posture Four: perform Movement **1** while walking forward.

Posture Five: perform Movement **2** while walking backward.

Flow Chart for the Basic E Tai Chi Sequence

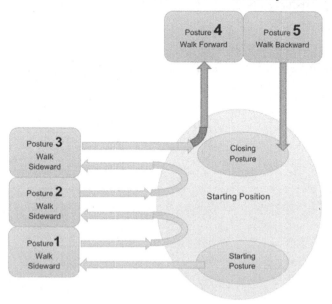

Starting Posture: perform **Movement 1** four times while **standing**.

Posture **One**: perform **Movement 1** while walking 4 steps **sideways** left and 4 steps right.

Posture **Two**: perform **Movement 2** while walking 4 steps **sideways** left and 4 steps right.

Posture **Three**: perform **Movement 3** while walking 4 steps **sideways** left and 4 steps right.

Posture **Four**: perform **Movement 1** while walking 4 steps **forward**.

Posture **Five**: perform **Movement 2** while walking 4 steps **backward**.

Closing Posture: perform **Movement 2** four times while **standing**.

.

Detailed Flow Chart for the Basic Level E Tai Chi Sequence

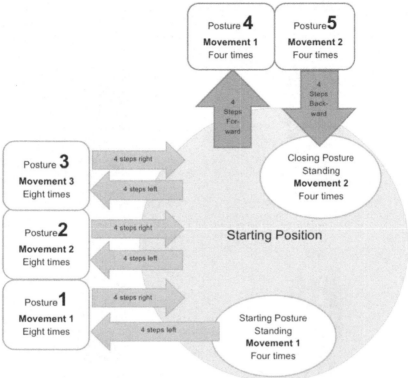

Starting Posture: perform **Movement 1** four times while **standing**.

Posture **One**: perform **Movement 1** while walking 4 steps **sideways** left and 4 steps right.

Posture **Two**: perform **Movement 2** while walking 4 steps **sideways** left and 4 steps right.

Posture **Three**: perform **Movement 3** while walking 4 steps **sideways** left and 4 steps right.

Posture **Four**: perform **Movement 1** while walking 4 steps **forward**.

Posture **Five**: perform **Movement 2** while walking 4 steps **backward**.

Closing Posture: perform **Movement 2** four times while **standing**.

Let us briefly review the basic hand/arm movements in E Tai Chi. See the details in Chapter 4.

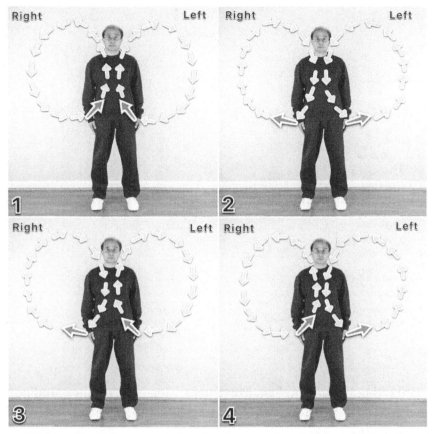

Photo #1. Movement 1: simultaneously circle your hands up through the midline of the body and circle your hands down and out to your sides (simultaneously circle your left hand counterclockwise and right hand clockwise).

Photo #2. Movement 2: simultaneously circle your hands up, out to your sides, and circle your hands down along the midline of the body (simultaneously circle your left hand clockwise and right hand counterclockwise).

Photo #3 and **Photo #4. Movement 3**: simultaneously circle your hands in the same direction (counterclockwise or clockwise) in front of the body.

Starting Posture

This posture is similar to the **Commencing** posture in most of the Tai Chi styles and many qigong exercises. In traditional Tai Chi Commencing, you raise and drop your hands just in front of your torso. Your hands circle down outward to the sides of the body in E Tai Chi.

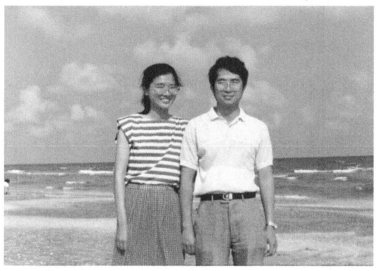

Starting Posture: Perform Movement 1 **four** times while standing.

Flow Chart for Starting Postures
(Perform Movement 1 while standing.)

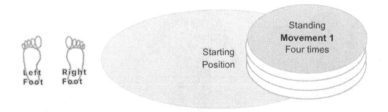

Stand naturally in a relaxed state with feet shoulder-width apart. Your hands and arms hang loosely at your sides. Bend your knees to 10-20-degrees. Keep your eyes straight ahead. Breathe naturally and peacefully.

As you slowly raise your arms, slowly straighten your knee joints. When your hands descend, your torso will sink with gentle flexion of your knees and return to the starting posture. Then repeat the same movement three more times. The action is the same, as illustrated in **Figure 5-1** in Chapter 5.

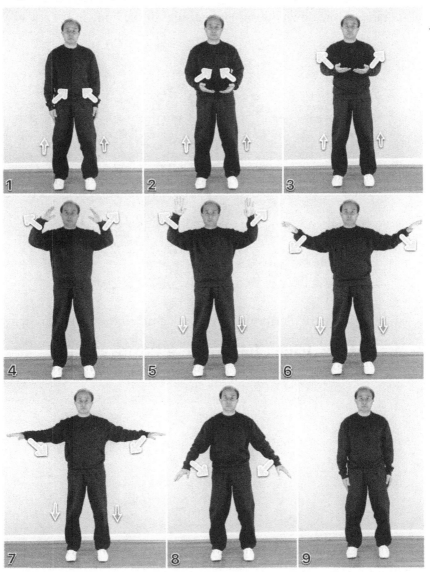

Figure 6-1A. Starting Posture: Standing Movement 1 (front view).

Key points for **Figure 6-1A**.

Photo #1: **Routine Stance**. Stand with feet shoulder-width apart. Your hands rest at your sides. The knees are flexed at 10-20 degrees. Keep your torso upright.

Photo #2: Slowly straighten your knee joints when you are raising your hands through the midline (**Movement 1**). The palms are directed upwards when the hands are ascending. The fingers of both hands point to each other diagonally. You look like you are holding a big ball in front of your body

Photo #3: The hands continue to ascend with the palms facing upward.

Photo #4: When your hands are raised above shoulder level, your palms gradually turn (pronate) to face inward during the transition from facing upward to facing forward.

Photo #5: As the hands are lifted above the head, the palms turn to face forward. You look like you are pushing the ball away.

Photo #6: Slowly bend your knee joints when dropping your hands to the sides. The palms face downward when the hands are descending.

Photo #7: The hands continue to descend. They are at shoulder level at this moment. Continue to sink your body and bend your knees gently.

Photo #8: The hands are returning to your sides.

Photo #9: The hands have returned to your sides. You are back to **Routine Stance**.

The Important Point

Bend your knees to a lesser degree or do not flex your knees at all if you feel uncomfortable or pain in Routine Stance or Transitional Stance.

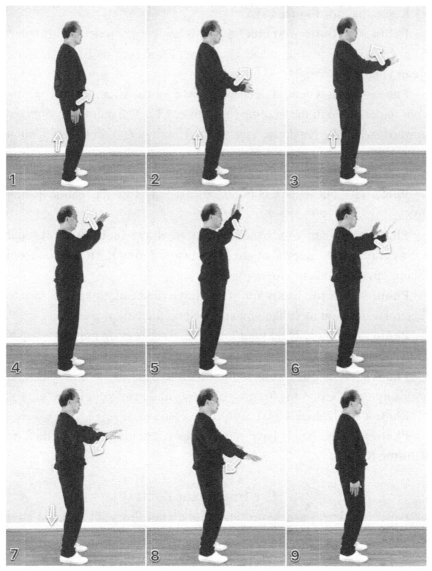

Figure 6-1B. Starting Posture: Standing Movement 1 (lateral view).

Posture One: The Sun Creeping Up

In Posture One, walk four steps sideward to the left and then walk four steps sideward right back to the starting location while doing **Movement 1**. Posture One is like the action of holding and lifting a ball. The escalating ball looks like the sun that is rising slowly.

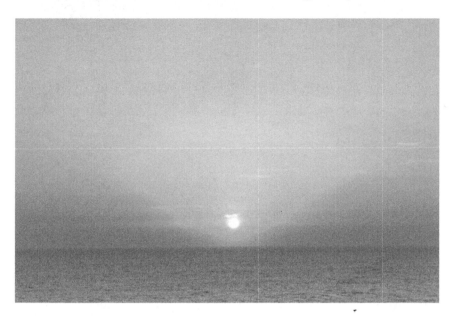

Let us briefly review the execution of walking sideways. See the details in Chapter 3.

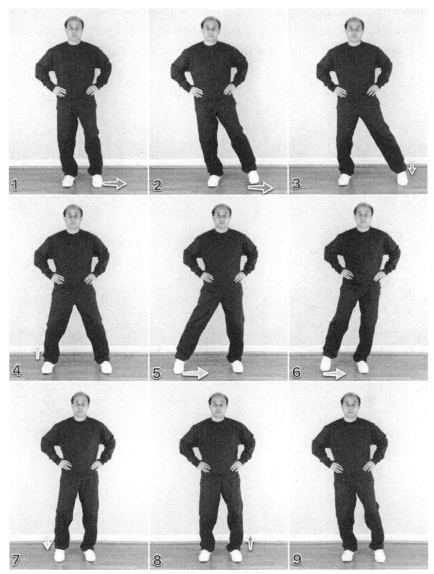

Figure 6-2A. Walking sideways.

Key points for **Figure 6-2A**.

Photo #1: **Routine Stance** to **Transitional Stance**. Stand with feet shoulder-width apart. The knees are flexed at 10-20 degrees. Keep both feet pointed forward during walking sideways. Shift your body weight to the right leg. Lift the left heel up and get ready to step out.

Photo #2: Take a step sideways left with the left foot.

Photo #3: The toes of the left foot touch the ground.

Photo #4: Gradually shift the body weight to the left leg. At this moment, the weight is evenly distributed between both legs.

Photo #5: The body weight is fully shifted to the left leg with the right heel off the ground. You are ready to bring your right foot in.

Photo #6: Move the right foot toward the left foot.

Photo #7: The right foot comes in contact with the ground. The toes of the right foot touch the ground first. You are in **Transitional Stance** (the left leg is the supporting leg).

Photo #8: Gradually shift the body weight to the right leg. At this moment, the weight is evenly distributed between both legs. You are back to **Routine Stance**.

Photo #9: After having transferred all your weight back to the right leg, you are in **Transitional Stance** again (the right leg is the supporting leg). You are ready to take the second sideward step with the left foot.

If you want to walk sideways to the right, then you can start by taking a step sideways right with the right foot in the same way as described above.

The Important Point

Bend your knees to a lesser degree or do not flex your knees at all if you feel uncomfortable or pain in Routine Stance or Transitional Stance.

Posture One: Walk **four** steps sideways to the left and perform Movement 1 **four** times, and then walk **four** steps sideways to the right and perform Movement 1 **four** times.

Flow Chart for Posture One

(Perform Movement 1 while walking sideways.)

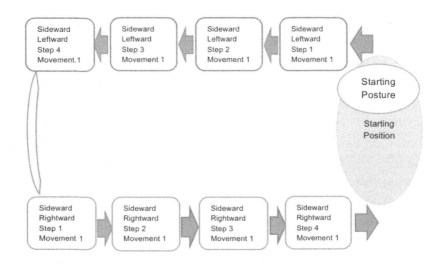

Flow Chart for Sideway Walking Steps

Walking Leftward

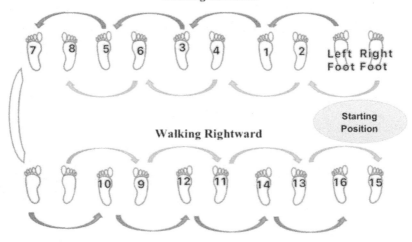

Walking Rightward

The numbers in the foot diagram indicate the step sequence.

The execution of **Posture One**.

You are in **Routine Stance** after Starting Posture. Stand with feet shoulder-width apart. The knees are flexed at 10-20 degrees. Shift your body weight to the right leg, and you are back in **Transitional Stance** (the right leg is the supporting leg). As you start to circle your hands up through the midline to perform Movement 1, step out to the left with your left foot and, at the same time, gradually shift the body weight to the left leg. Be sure to make an easy sideward step. The distance between your two feet is one to two feet wide. The toes of the feet keep facing forward.

As in regular sideways walking, when you start to take a side step, lift the heel of the moving foot off the ground first and then the whole foot. The toes of the sideward-moving foot touch the ground first. The above principle applies to all the sideward-moving postures (Postures One, Two, and Three).

As you start to drop your arms to the sides, bring the right foot in and shift the body weight back to the right leg. You will notice: when a leg sustains the body weight, the knee joint on the same side of the leg will be in the mildly flexed position. The body weight shifts from right to left and then from left to right alternately and continuously while you are performing the hand movements. Repeat the same movement three more times.

In summary, make a side step to the left with the left foot when you circle your hands up, and then move the right foot in toward the left foot as your hands are descending.

After you have finished the last leftward Movement 1, simultaneously circle your hands up through the midline and walk to the right in the same way as you perform the leftward Movement 1.

In other words, when you circle your hands up, take a side step right with your right foot, and gradually shift your weight to the right leg. When your hands are going down, bring the left foot in and progressively shift your bodyweight back to the left leg. Repeat the same movements three more times until you return to the starting location.

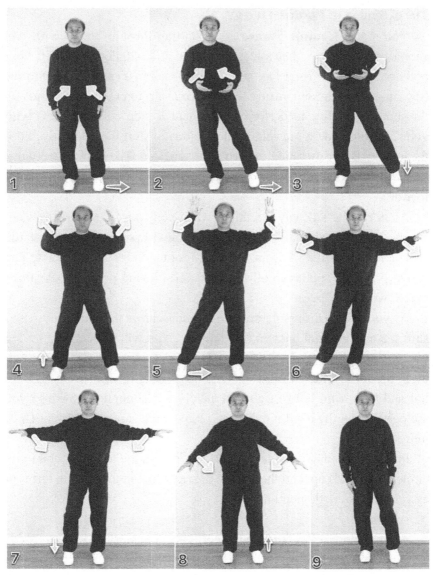

Figure 6-2B: Posture One: perform Movement 1 and walk sideways to the **left**.

Key points for **Figure 6-2B.**
Walking sideways leftward while performing Movement 1.

Photo #1: **Routine Stance** to **Transitional Stance**. Stand with feet shoulder-width apart. The knees are flexed at 10-20 degrees. Shift your body weight to the right leg. Lift the left heel up and get ready to step out.

Photo #2: Take a step out leftward with your left foot when you are raising your hands along the midline (**Movement 1**).

Photo #3: Finish stepping out to the left with the toes of the left foot touching the ground.

Photo #4: Gradually shift your body weight to the left leg. At this moment, the body weight is evenly distributed between your legs.

Photo #5: As your hands are raised overhead, the body weight is entirely shifted to the left leg, and the right heel comes off the ground. Your palms face forward. You are ready to bring the right foot toward the left foot and circle your hands down to the sides.

Photo #6: Move the right foot closer to the left foot while you are lowering your hands.

Photo #7: The toes of the right foot come in contact with the ground. Now, you are back in **Transitional Stance** (the left leg is the supporting leg).

Photo #8: The hands continue to descend. Gradually shift your body weight to the right leg. At this moment, the body weight is evenly distributed between your legs. You are back in **Routine Stance**.

Photo #9: As your hands are returning to your sides, transfer your weight back to the right leg. You are in **Transitional Stance** again (the right leg is the supporting leg) and ready to take the second sideward step with the left foot. Repeat the same movement three more times.

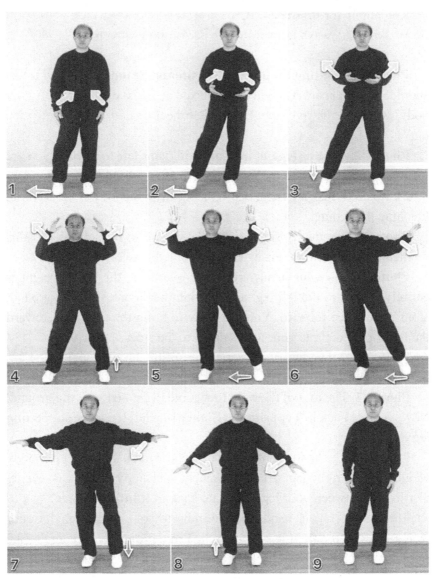

Figure 6-2C. Posture One: perform Movement 1 and walk sideways to the **right**.

You do not need to twist your torso when performing Posture One. In the beginning, you may simply walk sideways while performing hand movements without any coordination. As you have become familiar with the hand/foot movements, you will coordinate your hands and feet automatically. As I said before, any coordination is fine if you feel good. There are no absolute rules.

Walk eight steps sideways in each of the sideway postures. Of course, you can take as many steps as you like. The flowchart for sideways walking can be used in all the sideway postures.

Posture Two: Seagull Flying High

In Posture Two, walk four steps sideward to the left and then walk four steps sideward right back to the starting position while doing **Movement 2**. You look like a seagull that is hovering in the sky.

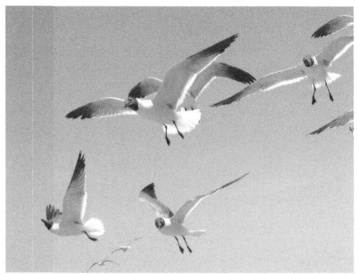

Posture Two: Walk **four** steps sideways to the left and perform Movement 2 **four** times, and then walk **four** steps sideways to the right and perform Movement 2 **four** times.

Flow Chart for Posture Two

(Perform Movement 2 while walking sideways.)

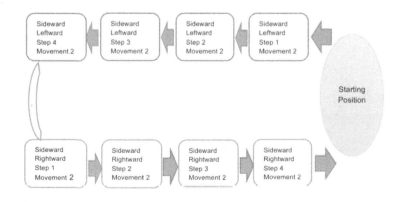

The execution of **Posture Two**.

You are back in **Transitional Stance** (the right leg is the supporting leg) after you have finished Posture One. As you start to circle your hands up to the sides to perform Movement 2, step out to the left with your left foot and, at the same time, gradually shift your body weight to the left leg. When you start to drop your arms through the midline, move the right foot in and shift the body weight back to the right leg. Your body weight shifts from right to left and then from left to right alternately and continuously while you are performing the hand movements. Repeat the same action three more times.

In summary, make a side step to the left with the left foot when you circle your hands up, and then move the right foot toward the left foot as your hands are descending.

After you have finished the last leftward Movement 2, circle your hands up to the sides and walk sideways to the right in the same way as you perform the leftward Movement 2. Repeat the same movements four times until you return to the starting location.

Flow Chart for Sideway Walking Steps

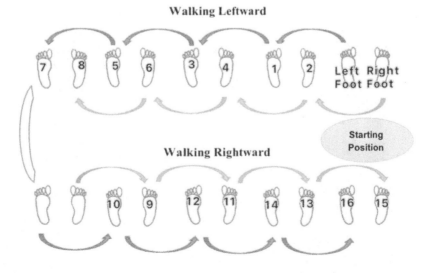

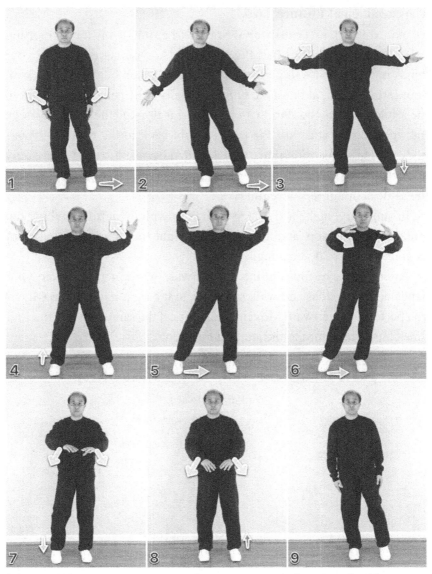

Figure 6-3A. Posture Two: perform Movement 2 and walk sideways to the **left**.

Key points for **Figure 6-3A.**

Walking sideways leftward while performing Movement 2.

Photo #1: At the conclusion of Posture One, you are back in **Transitional Stance**. Standing with the right foot supporting the body and the left foot placed parallel to the supporting leg. You are ready to step out.

Photo #2: Take a step sideward left when you are raising your hands to the sides (**Movement 2**).

Photo #3: The toes of the left foot are touching the ground.

Photo #4: Gradually shift your body weight to the left leg. At this moment, the body weight is evenly distributed between both legs.

Photo #5: As your hands are raised overhead, the body weight is entirely shifted to the left leg, and the right heel comes off the ground. Your palms face forward. You are ready to bring the right foot toward the left foot and circle your hands down through the midline.

Photo #6: Move the right foot toward the left foot while you are lowering your hands.

Photo #7: The toes of the right foot come in contact with the ground. Now, you are back in **Transitional Stance** (the left leg is the supporting leg).

Photo #8: Gradually shift your body weight to the right leg. At this moment, the body weight is evenly distributed between both legs. You are back to **Routine Stance**.

Photo #9: As your hands are returning to your sides, transfer your weight back to the right leg. You are in **Transitional Stance** again (the right leg is the supporting leg) and ready to take the second sideward step with the left foot. Repeat the same movement three more times.

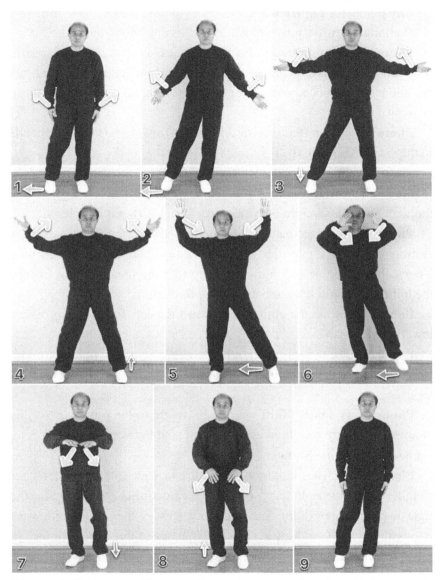

Figure 6-3B. Posture Two: perform Movement 2 and walk sideways to the **right**.

Posture Three: Performing Yangge Dance

In Posture Three, walk four steps sideward to the left and then walk four steps sideward right back to the starting location while doing Movement 3: simultaneously circle both hands counterclockwise (to the left) and clockwise (to the right). What you are doing is like performing Yangge dance. (For more details on this topic, see *Wikipedia: Yangge*.)

Yangge Dance is a Chinese folk dance characterized by twisting the body and waving hands rhythmically. Only Zhaobao-style Tai Chi has some similar movements. But the names of those movements do not fit the features of Posture Three. Therefore, I coin Posture Three as **"Performing Yangge Dance."**

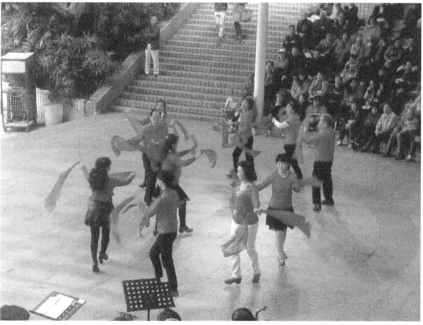

Retirees are performing Yangge Dance in Yuexiu Park in Guangzhou, China.

Posture Three: Walk **four** steps sideways to the left and perform Movement 3 **four** times, and then walk **four** steps sideways to the right and perform Movement 3 **four** times.

Flow Chart for Posture Three
(Perform Movement 3 while walking sideways.)

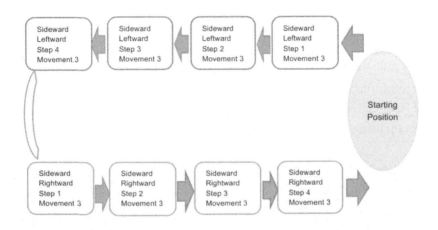

Flow Chart for Sideway Walking Steps
Walking Leftward

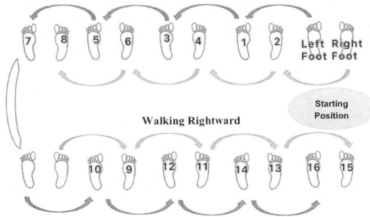

Walking Rightward

The execution of **Posture Three**.

At the conclusion of Posture Two, you are back in **Transitional Stance** (the right leg is the supporting leg). You are ready to perform the leftward Movement 3 (simultaneously circle both hands counterclockwise). Step out to the left with your left foot and, at the same time, gradually shift the body weight to the left leg. When you start to drop your arms, move the right foot toward the left foot and shift the bodyweight back to the right leg. Your body weight shifts from right to left and then from left to right alternately and continuously while you are performing the leftward Movement 3. Repeat the same movement three more times.

In summary, make a step with the left foot to the left when you circle your hands up, and then bring your right foot in as your hands are descending.

After you have finished the last leftward Movement 3, simultaneously circle your hands clockwise and walk sideways to the right in the same way as you perform the leftward Movement 3. Repeat the same movements four times until you return to the starting position.

You do not need to twist your torso when performing Posture Three. In the beginning, you may simply walk sideways while playing the hand movements without any coordination.

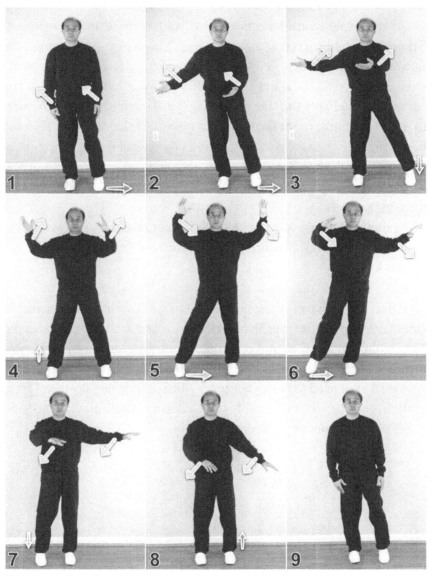

Figure 6-4A. Posture Three: perform the leftward Movement 3 and walk sideways to the **left**.

Key points for **Figure 6-4A**:

Walk sideways to the left while performing the leftward Movement 3.

Photo #1: At the conclusion of Posture Two, you are back in **Transitional Stance**. Standing with the right foot supporting the body and the left foot placed parallel to the supporting leg.

Photo #2: Take a step sideward left when you are circling your hands counterclockwise (the leftward **Movement 3**).

Photo #3: The toes of the left foot are touching the ground.

Photo #4: Gradually shift your body weight to the left leg. At this moment, the body weight is evenly distributed between both legs.

Photo #5: As your hands are raised overhead, the body weight is entirely shifted to the left leg, and the right heel comes off the ground. Your palms face forward. You are ready to bring the right foot toward the left foot and circle your hands down.

Photo #6: Move the right foot toward the left foot while you are lowering your hands.

Photo #7: The toes of the right foot come in contact with the ground. Now, you are back in **Transitional Stance** (the left leg is the supporting leg).

Photo #8: The hands continue to descend. Gradually shift your body weight to the right leg. At this moment, the body weight is evenly distributed between both legs. You are back to **Routine Stance**.

Photo #9: As your hands are returning to your sides, transfer your weight back to the right leg. You are in **Transitional Stance** again (the right leg is the supporting leg) and ready to take the second sideward step with the left foot. Repeat the same movement three more times.

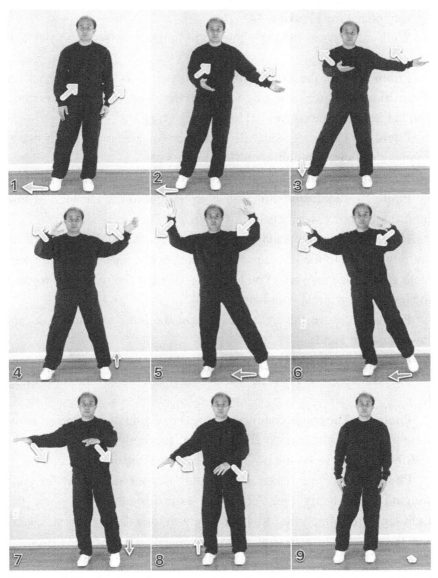

Figure 6-4B. Posture Three: perform the rightward Movement 3 and walk sideways to the **right**.

Posture Four: Swimming on Land

Walking forward while performing Movement 1 looks like swimming breaststroke on land.

In short, when you circle your hands up through the midline, step out forward with one foot. When you drop your hands to your sides, move the other foot (the back foot) forward and place it parallel to the front foot. See the following flowchart.

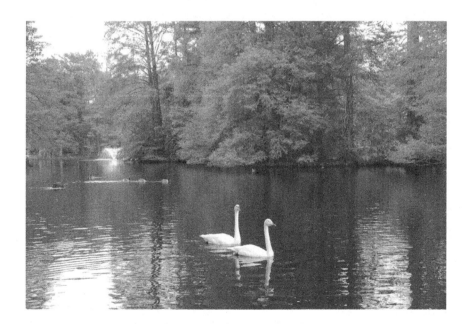

Posture Four: Walk **four** steps forward and perform Movement 1 **four** times.

Flow Chart of Posture Four
(Perform Movement 1 while walking forward.)

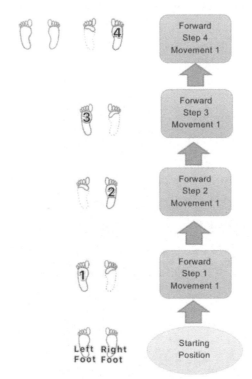

The execution of **Posture Four**. See **Figure 6-5A** and **Figure 6-5B**.

After having completed Posture Three, you return to your original starting position. You are back in **Transitional Stance**: the right leg is supporting the bodyweight with the toes of the left foot touching the ground.

Lift your left foot and step forward while raising your hands through the midline to perform Movement 1. As you do during normal walking, when starting to take a step, lift the heel of the moving foot off the ground first and then the whole foot. The heel of the forward-moving foot touches the ground first. The above principle applies to all the forward postures.

As your hands circle up above the head (to any height you like), gradually sink the torso and shift the body weight from the right leg to the left leg. The left foot will be in complete contact with the ground. Now you realize that you are taking a small bow stance with the left knee slightly bent in front and the right leg straight behind you. Seventy percent of the body weight should be distributed to the front foot and 30 % to the rear foot.

When you start to descend the hands to the sides, gradually shift the entire weight of your body to the left leg (the front leg) and slowly lift the right heel off the ground. When your hands are lowered to shoulder level, swing the right leg forward. Remember, the left leg is supporting the whole-body weight during the swing of the right leg.

Your right foot will be positioned next to the left foot when the hands return to your sides. Gently place the toes of the right foot on the ground. This is the same position as the beginning position except that the left leg supports the body here. Now you have returned to **Transitional Stance**. Alternatively, you can skip **Transitional Stance** and continue the forward step without touching the ground if you have strong legs.

Then, go on to take the second step with the right foot while raising your hands again to perform the next Movement 1. Repeat the same action as above. The difference is that you take a right forward step.

Here, you circle your hands up and down while walking forward. You look like you are swimming breaststroke on land. Remember, it is a normal walking step at a slower pace. Your step length should be similar to the one during your regular walking. You should take comfortable steps to avoid knee pain or injury.

Repeat the left forward step and the right forward step one more time while playing Movement 1. Perform Movement 1 four times and take a total of four forward steps. Nevertheless, you can play them as many times as you like. When you finish the last Movement 1, you are back in **Transitional Stance** with the right leg supporting the body weight. Now you are ready to go on to Posture Five.

In summary, when you raise your hands along the midline, step forward with one foot. When you drop the hands to your sides, step forward with another foot. The coordination of circular hand movements and slow walking steps maintain the fluidity and continuity of traditional

Tai Chi. However, in the beginning, you can just walk naturally while performing the hand movements without any coordination.

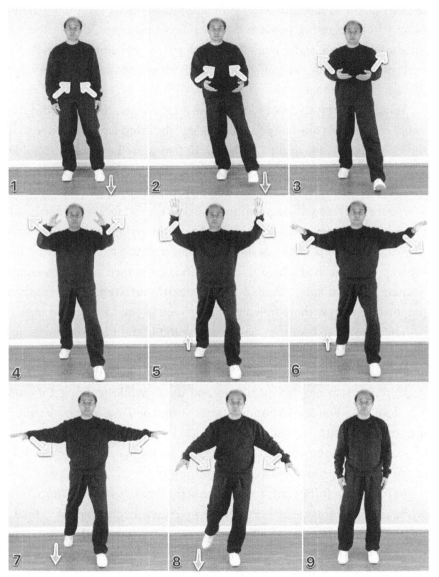

Figure 6-5A. Posture Four, the first step (front view)

Key points for **Figure 6-5A** and **Figure 6-5B**.

Photo #1: You have finished the last rightward Movement 3 with your hands at your sides. You are in **Transitional Stance** with the right leg supporting the body weight.

Photo #2: Step forward with your left foot while circling your hands up through the midline with the palms facing upward (**Movement 1**).

Photo #3: The left heel is touching the ground while you continue to raise your hands.

Photo #4: Your hands continue to ascend. As the left foot comes in complete contact with the ground, gradually shift your weight to the left leg.

Photo #5: The hands are raised above the head with the palms facing forward. Now you are in **Bow Stance** with the front knee (left knee) mildly flexed and the back leg (the right leg) straight.

When shifting the body weight from the right leg to the left leg, you should use the back leg (here the right leg) to push the body forward so that the front lower leg (here the left leg) forms a 90-degree angle relative to the front foot or the ground. This is a typical **bow stance** in Chinese martial arts. When **you drive the body forward by the back leg**, the front knee joint will not be over-flexed.

Photo #6: As you are circling your hands down to the sides, gradually shift your entire weight to the left leg with the right heel off the ground.

Photo #7: After the body weight has been completely transferred to the left leg, you are ready to take a step forward with your right foot. Your hands are at shoulder level at this moment.

Photo #8: The right leg is swinging forward while the hands continue to descend.

Photo #9: Your hands have returned to your sides when your right foot becomes parallel to the left foot. The toes of the right foot gently touch the ground while the left foot continues to support the body. Now you are back in **Transitional Stance.** You are ready to continue the forward step with the right foot and proceed to perform the next Movement 1.

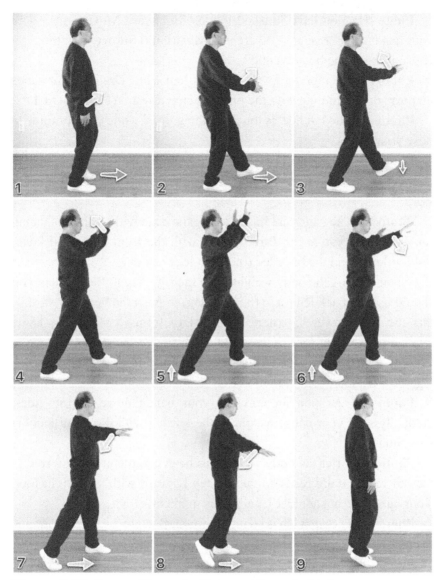

Figure 6-5B. Posture Four, the first step (lateral view).

The Important Point

Bend your front knee to a lesser degree and take shorter steps if you feel uncomfortable or pain in Bow Stance.

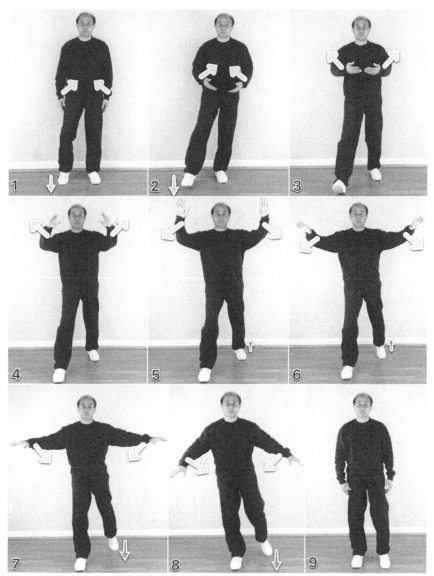

Figure 6-5C. Posture Four, the second step (front view).

Figure 6-5C and **Figure 6-5D** show the second step in Posture Four. You do the same thing as in **Figure 6-5A** and **Figure 6-5B,** except you step forward with the right foot instead of the left foot. Repeat the same action with your left foot and right foot one more time, respectively. Walk four steps forward and perform Movement 1 four times in Posture Four.

149

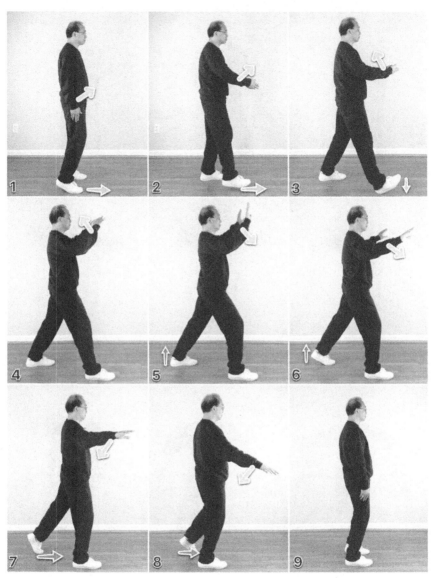

Figure 6-5D. Posture Four, the second step (lateral view).

Posture Five: Swan Spreading Its Wings

Walking backward while performing Movement 2.

This posture is similar to **White Crane Spread Its Wings** (白鹤亮翅) in many styles of Tai Chi, where one hand moves down to the side while another hand rises above the head. In E Tai Chi Posture Five, you imitate a swan spreading its wings because both your hands ascend simultaneously.

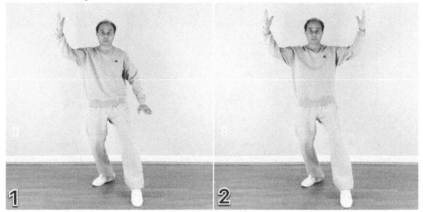

Photo #1: White Crane Spread Its Wings in traditional Tai Chi.
Photo #2: Swan Spreading Its Wings in E Tai Chi.

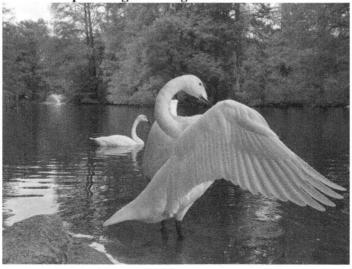

Posture Five: Walk **four** steps backward and perform Movement 2 **four** times.

Flow Chart of Posture Five

(Perform Movement 2 while walking backward.)

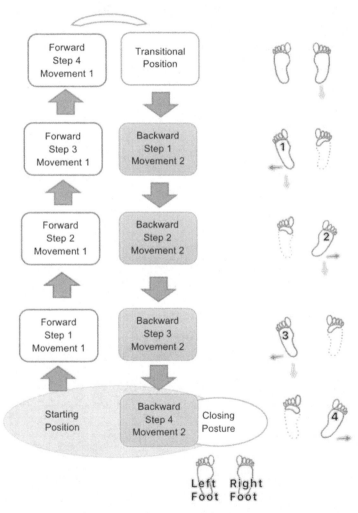

Let us practice **Posture Five**.

At the conclusion of Posture Four, you are back in **Transitional Stance** with the right leg supporting the body weight. Then circularly spread the hands outward (**Movement 2**) as you raise your left foot and step backward. The toes of your left foot touch the ground first, and then the whole foot plants on the ground as the body weight is gradually transferred to the left leg (the rear leg). It is a natural backward step that is slowed down. Make sure not to stride too long. Otherwise, you can hurt your knee joints.

As in regular backward walking, when you start to take a step backward, lift the heel of the backward-moving foot off the ground first and then the whole foot. The toes of the backward-moving foot touch the ground first. This principle applies to all the backward-moving postures.

The left heel will be naturally moved inward as the whole foot contacts the ground, and the body weight is gradually shifted to the left leg. The left foot (the rear foot) is angled outward at 35-45 degrees. The inward movement of the left heel should occur spontaneously because the resulting posture produces optimal body stability. The final posture is: the toes of the front foot (here the right foot) are pointed forward, and the rear foot is angled outward at 35-45 degrees. See Flow Chart and **Photos #3 and #4** in **Figure 6-6A** and **Figure 6-6B**.

Please make sure not to let the heel of the real foot cross the midline. The crossing of your feet will cause you to lose balance easily. As I mentioned, you do it right when you feel natural and comfortable.

As you continue to circle your hands up above shoulder level, shift all your weight to the left leg. In this position, the whole body is supported by the left leg (the rear leg), and the right foot (the front foot) will spontaneously shift backward a few inches with the right knee joint mildly flexed. This posture happens automatically because it produces optimal body stability and makes you feel comfortable. Now you are in **Empty Stance**. See **Photo #5** in **Figure 6-6A** and **Figure 6-6B**. When your hands are raised overhead, you feel like a swan that is spreading its wings.

Pull the right foot back as you start to circle the hands down through the midline. The right foot is positioned next to the left foot when the hands return to your sides. This is the same position as the beginning position except that the left leg supports the body here. You are in **Transitional Stance** again. You can gently place the toes of the right foot on the ground. Alternatively, continue your backward step without touching the ground and repeat the same action as above. The difference is that you take a step backward with the right foot.

As described above for walking backward with the left foot, the right foot is angled at 35-45 degrees outward when the whole right foot lands on the ground. The entire body weight is shifted to the rear leg (here the right leg) as your hands continue to ascend. At this moment, you will notice that the front heel (here the left foot) naturally moves outward during weight shifting. Consequently, the left knee is in line with the left foot. See Flow Chart and **Photo #2, Photo #3**, and **Photo #4** in **Figure 6-6C** and **Figure 6-6D**.

When your hands continue to arise, the left foot will spontaneously move backward a few inches as described above for the right foot. The final posture is: the toes of the left foot (the front foot) are pointed forward and the right foot (the rear foot) angled outward at 35-45 degrees. You are in **Empty Stance** again.

Remember: when you take the first backward step with the left foot, the right heel does not need to shift at all because the toes of the right foot are already pointed forward at the beginning of Posture Five.

Repeat the left backward step and the right backward step while playing Movement 2 one more time, respectively. Practice Movement 2 four times and take four steps backward.

When you finish the last Movement 2, the toes of your left foot are touching the ground, and your right foot is angled outward at 30-45 degrees, supporting the body weight. As you shift the body weight to the left leg, move the right heel outward so that the tip of the right foot will be pointed forward. Now, you have returned to the starting posture, **Routine Stance**. You can move on to perform Closing Posture. See **Figure 6-7A** (Transition from Posture Five to Closing) in the next section.

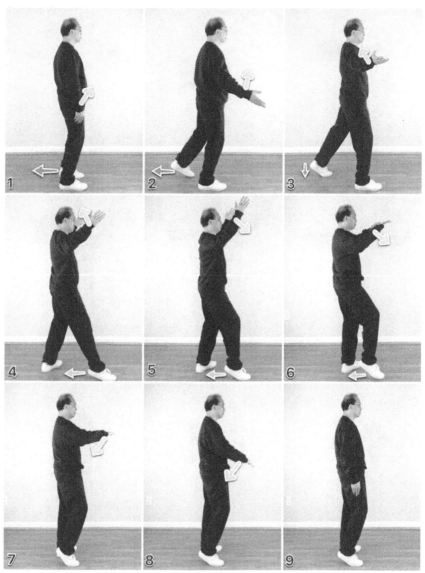

Figure 6-6B. Posture Five, the first backward step (lateral view). (**Figure 6-6A** is placed on the following page for convenience.)

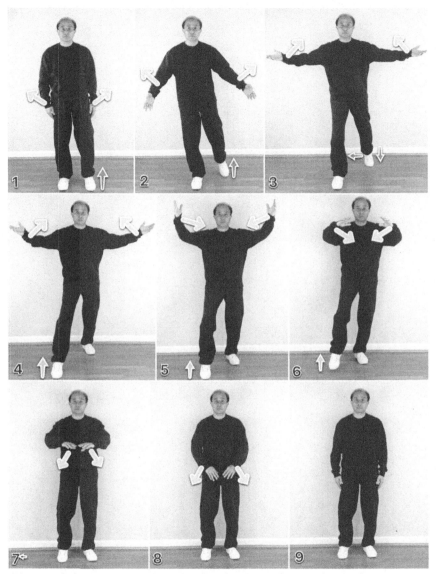

Figure 6-6A. Posture Five, the first backward step (front view).

Key points for **Figure 6-6A** and **Figure 6-6B**.

Photo #1: At the conclusion of Posture Four, you are back in **Transitional Stance** with the right leg supporting the body and ready to step back with your left foot.

Photo #2: Step backward with your left foot while circling your hands up to the sides (**Movement 2**).

156

Photo #3: As the toes of your left foot are touching the ground, gradually shift the weight to the left leg while you continue to raise your hands. The left heel will be naturally moved inward as the whole left foot contacts the ground. Both hands are at shoulder level.

Photo #4: Your left foot (the back foot) is in complete contact with the ground. The right heel (the front foot) comes off the ground as your weight has been entirely shifted to the left leg.

The toes of the right foot (the front foot) are pointed forward, and the left foot (the back foot) is angled outward at 35-45 degrees.

Photo #5: As your hands are raised overhead, your right foot spontaneously moves backward a few inches.

Now you are in **Empty Stance.** Stand with the rear leg (here the left leg) supporting the entire weight of the body. The back knee (here the left knee) is flexed at 10-20 degrees. The toes of the front foot (here the right foot) are placed in the front and pointed forward, and the rear foot (here the left foot) is angled outward at 35-45 degrees.

Photo #6: As you are circling your hands down through the midline of the body, slowly bring your right foot back.

Photo #7: The right foot is positioned parallel to the left foot with the toes of the right foot touching the ground.

Photo #8: Your hands continue to descend.

Photo #9: Your hands have returned to your sides. Now you are back in **Transitional Stance**: your left leg is supporting your weight while the toes of your right foot gently touch the ground to keep balance. You are ready to continue the backward step with the right foot and proceed to perform the next Movement 2. See **Figure 6-6C** and **Figure 6-6D**.

The Important Point

Bend your knees to a lesser degree or do not flex your knees at all if you feel uncomfortable or pain in Routine Stance, Transitional Stance, or Empty Stance.

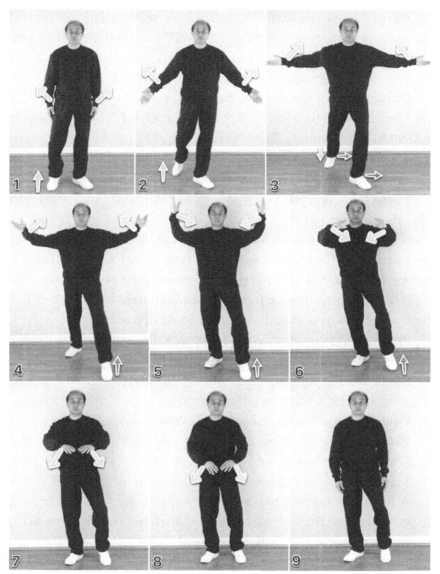

Figure 6-6C. Posture Five, the second backward step (front view).

Key points for **Figure 6-6C** and **Figure 6-6D.**

Take the second backward step with your right foot while performing Movement 2 in the same way as described in **Figure 6-6A.**

Photo #1: At the conclusion of the first backward Movement 2, you are back in **Transitional Stance** with the left leg supporting the body and ready to step back with your right foot.

Photo #2: Step backward with your right foot while circling your hands up to the sides (**Movement 2**).

Photo #3: As the toes of your right foot are touching the ground, gradually shift your weight to the right leg while you continue to raise your hands. The right heel will be naturally moved inward as the whole right foot contacts the ground.

Your left foot becomes the front foot and is angled at 30-45 degrees. Therefore, you need to move the left heel outward so that the left knee is in line with the left foot. (When you take the first backward step with your left foot, your right foot is already pointed forward. Therefore, you do not need to shift the right heel.)

Photo #4: The right foot (the back foot) is in complete contact with the ground. The left heel (the front foot) comes off the ground as your weight has been entirely shifted to the right leg.

The toes of the left foot are pointed forward, and the right foot (the rear foot) is angled outward at 35-45 degrees.

Photo #5: As your hands are raised overhead, your left foot spontaneously moves backward a few inches. Now you are in **Empty Stance**.

Photo #6: As you are circling your hands down through the midline of the body, slowly bring the left foot back.

Photo #7: The left foot is positioned parallel to the right foot with the toes of the left foot touching the ground.

Photo #8: Your hands continue to descend.

Photo #9: Your hands have returned to your sides. Now you are back in **Transitional Stance**: your right leg is supporting your weight while the toes of your left foot gently touch the ground to maintain balance. You are ready to continue the backward step with the left foot and proceed to perform the next Movement 2.

You will carry out the same action when taking the third and fourth backward steps. In Posture Five, practice Movement 2 four times and take four steps backward.

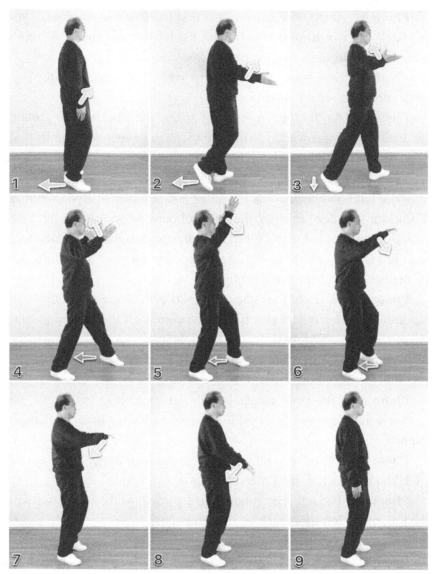

Figure 6-6D. Posture Five, the second backward step (lateral view).

Closing Posture

This posture is nothing new: Perform **Movement 2** four times while standing, as described in Chapter 5. We are done!

Stand naturally in a relaxed state with feet shoulder-width apart. Your hands and arms hang loosely at your sides. Bend your knees to 10-20-degrees. As you circle your arms up to the sides (**Movement 2**), slowly straighten your knee joints. When your hands descend through the midline of the body, your torso will sink with gentle flexion of the knees and return to the starting posture. Then repeat the same movement three more times.

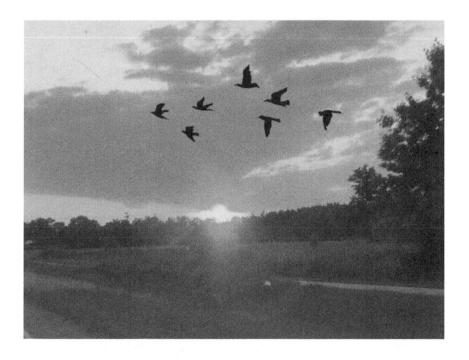

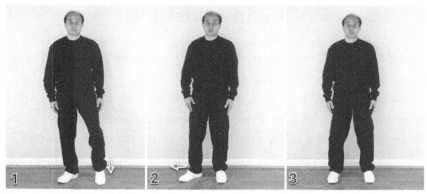

Figure 6-7A Transition from Posture Five to Closing Posture.

Photo #1: At the conclusion of Posture Five, your right foot is angled at 30-45 degrees. Your right leg is supporting your weight while the toes of your left foot gently touch the ground to maintain balance.

Photo #2: Shift your weight to the left leg and move the right heel outward to bring your feet parallel to each other.

Photo #3: Distribute your weight evenly between both legs. Now you are back in **Routine Stance** and ready to proceed Closing Posture.

Closing Posture: Perform Movement 2 **four** times while standing.

Flow Chart for Closing Posture

(Perform Movement 2 while standing.)

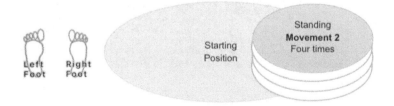

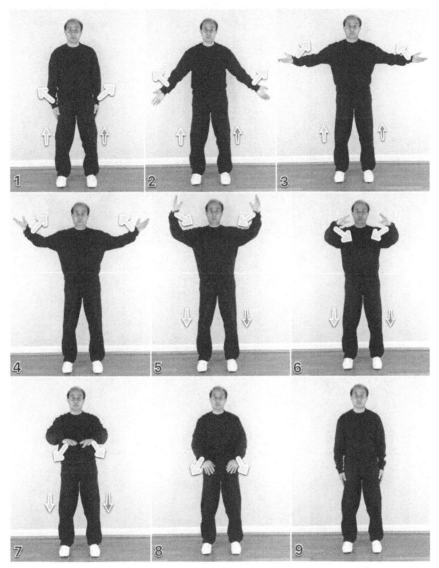

Figure 6-7B. Closing Posture: Perform Movement 2 while standing (front view).

Practice Standing Movement 2

Straighten your knees when circling your hands and arms up to the sides. Gently sink your torso and flex your knees when your hands circle down through the midline.

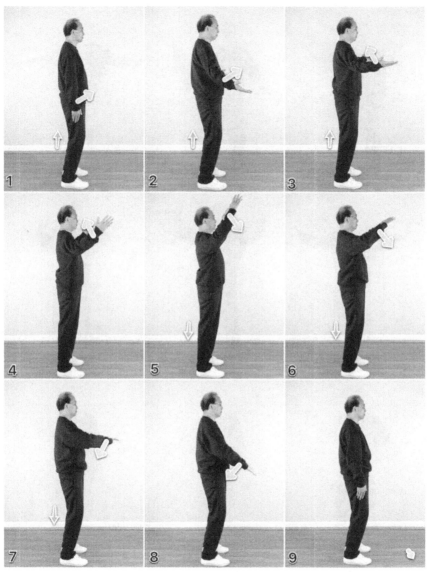

Figure 6-7C. Closing Posture: Perform Movement 2 while standing (lateral view).

Epilog

"授人以鱼，不如授之以渔，授人以鱼只救一时之急，授人以渔则可解一生之需。"

Give a man a fish, and you feed him for a day. Teach him how to fish, and you feed him for a lifetime.

—Chinese Proverb

As I mentioned earlier, you can perform the E Tai Chi hand/arm movements in any direction. Moreover, your hands or arms can be overlapped (crossed over the midline of your body) and moved in large or small circles as long as you feel good. Again, there is no strict rule in E Tai Chi. You are doing the right thing if you practice it gently, comfortably, and safely. E Tai Chi is for your personal health only, not for fighting or competition.

Congratulations!

After you have finished reading this book, you will obtain a valuable tool, E Tai Chi, at hand, which you can use and perfect anytime and anywhere. You can create your own E Tai Chi sequence by using the six hand movements and different ways of walking or standing. You make it, own it, and enjoy it! It will help you keep healthy, achieve peace of mind, cultivate the happiness of feeling good, and have a smile all the time. Whatever exercise you do, you should do it moderately, safely, and regularly.

Where there is a smile, there is a chance, peace, and happiness.
— Quoted from my book: ***Life and Medicine***.

Acknowledgments

I am very grateful to the following people who helped make this book a reality.

Jo, my beautiful wife, has read my book many times, comes up with many bright ideas, and continues to make caustic and funny remarks. She has taken many wonderful photos and become my first E Tai Chi student. At present, she is translating the book into Chinese. I hope that the Chinese version of the book will be published later this year. Her support and love have made my life meaningful.

Lisa Bozik, MD, my colleague, proofread two chapters of the book, provided critical comments, and corrected my English grammar errors.

The clinic staff support my work every day and are interested in E Tai Chi. Some of them participated in taking the gorgeous picture on Page 5. They are Trista Bonnette, Carolyn Dewitt, Kayla Easterlin, Ashley Harris, Jami Odom, Deidre Oliver, Melanie Sheppard, and Charlotte Shuler.

Some of my patients put up with my Tai Chi teaching during office visits.

About the Author

Dr. Yongxin Li, the inventor of E Tai Chi, graduated from Guangzhou Medical College (Guangzhou Medical University) in China in the 1980s. He came to the U.S. in 1986 and received his Ph.D. degree in physiology from the University of Texas Medical Branch at Galveston in 1991. He completed his internal medicine residency at Wright State University School of Medicine in Dayton, Ohio in the 1990s. Since then, he has been practicing internal medicine in a southern state. Dr. Yongxin Li is the author of *Life and Medicine*: *Every Patient Teaches a Lesson*.

References

ACE Physical Therapy and Sports Medicine Institute. (2015, October 30). *Side Stepping to Treat Low Back and Lower Extremity Injuries.* Retrieved June 26, 2016, from ACE Physical Therapy and Sports Medicine Institute: http://www.ace-pt.org/2015/10/30/ace-physical-therapy-and-sports-medicine-institute-side-stepping-to-treat-low-back-and-lower-extremity-injuries/

Broad, W. J. (2012). The Science of Yoga The Risks and the Rewards.

Bryant, M. S., Workman, C. D., Hou, J.-G. G., Henson, H. K., & York, M. K. (2016). Acute and Long-Term Effects of Multidirectional Treadmill Training on Gait and Balance in Parkinson Disease. *PM R, 8*(12), 1151-1158.

Dicharry, J. (2010). Kinematics and kinetics of gait: from lab to clinic. *Clin Sports Med, 29*(3), 347-64.

Gilchrist, L. (1998). Age-related changes in the ability to side-step during gait. *Clin Biomech*, 91-97.

Handford, M. L., & Srinivasan, M. (2014). Sideways walking: preferred is slow, slow is optimal, and optimal is expensive. *Biol Lett., 10*(1), 20131006.

Hempel, S., Taylor, S. L., R, S. M., Miake-Lye, I. M., Beroes, J. M., Shanman, R., & Shekelle, P. G. (2014). *Evidence Map of Tai Chi.* Washington (DC): Department of Veterans Affairs (US).

Kim, T.-W., & Kim, Y.-W. (2014). Treadmill Sideways Gait Training with Visual Blocking for Patients with Brain Lesions. *J Phys Ther Sci., 26* (9), 1415–1418.

Lear, S., Gasevic, D., & Hu, W. (2016). The effect of overall and types of physical activity on mortality and cardiovascular events in 17 countries: Results from the Prospective Urban Rural Epidemiologic (PURE) study. *World*

Congress of Cardiology & Cardiovascular Health, (p. Abstract OC01_02). Mexico City, Mexico.

Li, Y. (2015). *Life and Medicine.* Amazon Digital Services LLC.

Li 李, D. (2003). *太极拳规范教程 The Textbook of Standardized Taijiquan.* 人民体育出版社.

Maki, B. E., & McIlroy, W. E. (2006). Control of rapid limb movements for balance recovery: age-related changes and implications for fall prevention. *Age Ageing, 35* (Suppl), ii12-ii18.

Men 门, H. (2011). *东岳太极拳 (Dongyue Taijiquan).* 人民体育出版社.

Mourdoukoutas, P. (2012, 1 14). *The Ten Golden Rules on Living the Good Life.* Retrieved 8 20, 2016, from Forbes.com: http://www.forbes.com/sites/panosmourdoukoutas/2012/01/14/the-ten-golden-rules-on-living-the-good-life/#21ac926a5c82

Nahin, R. L., Boineau, R., Khalsa, P. S., Stussman, B. J., & Weber, W. J. (2016). Evidence-Based Evaluation of Complementary Health Approaches for Pain Management in the United States. *Mayo Clinic Proceedings, 91*(9), 1292–1306.

Penman, S., M, C., P, S., & S, J. (2012). Yoga in Australia: Results of a national survey. *Int J Yoga, 5*(2), 92-101.

Rose, J. (n.d.). *Clinical Gait Analysis.* Retrieved 8 28, 2016, from https://web.stanford.edu/class/engr110/2009/Rose-08a.pdf

The United States Department of Veterans Affairs. (n.d.). *Clinical Staff Guide to Pedometers - Move!* Retrieved 8 28, 2016, from http://www.move.va.gov/docs/Resources/ClinicalStaffGuideToPedometer2011.pdf

The University of Washington. (n.d.). *Gait I: Overview, Overall Measures, and Phases of Gait.* Retrieved 8 28, 2016, from courses.washington.edu/.:

http://courses.washington.edu/anatomy/KinesiologySylla
bus/GaitPhasesKineticsKinematics.pdf

Wang, C., Schmid, C. H., Iversen, M. D., Harvey, W. F., Fielding, R. A., Driban, J. B., . . . McAli, T. (2016). Comparative Effectiveness of Tai Chi Versus Physical Therapy for Knee Osteoarthritis: A Randomized Trial. *Ann Intern Med, 165*(2), 77-86.

Wayne, P. M., & Fuerst, M. L. (2013). *The Harvard Medical School Guide to Tai Chi: 12 Weeks to a Healthy Body, Strong Heart, and Sharp Mind (Harvard Health Publications) Kindle Edition.* Shambhala Publications.

Wayne, P. M., Berkowitz, D. L., Litrownik, D. E., Buring, E, J., & Yeh, G. Y. (2014). What do we really know about the safety of tai chi?: A systemic review of adverse event reports in randomized trials. *Arch Phys Med Rehabil*, 2477-83.

Yan, J., Gu, W., Sun, J., Zhang, W., Li, B., & Pan, L. (2013). Efficacy of Tai Chi on pain, stiffness and function in patients with osteoarthritis: a meta-analysis. *PLoS One, 8*(4), e61672.

Yuan 苑, X. (2014). *成都市区太极拳练习者膝关节痛现状的调查与分析 (A Study of Knee Pain in Taijiquan Practitioners in Chengdu, China).* Retrieved 9 4, 2016, from 中国知网 (cnki): http://cdmd.cnki.com.cn/Article/CDMD-10653-1014364342.htm

Zeng, Y., Luo, T., Xie, H., Huang, M., & Cheng, A. (2014). Health benefits of qigong or tai chi for cancer patients: a systematic review and meta-analyses. *Complement Ther Med, 22*((1)), 173-86.

Zhu, D., Li, L., Qiu, P., Wang, S., Xie, Y., & Chen, X. (2011). 上海市区太极拳练习者膝关节疼痛调查分析 (A Survey on Knee Pain of Tai Chi Quan Practitioners in Shanghai Urban Area). *中国运动医学杂志 (Chin J Sports Med), 30*(9), 825-829.

Made in the USA
Monee, IL
10 December 2021